Sajeesh Kumar Bruce E. Dunn (Eds.)

Telepathology

Sajeesh Kumar   Bruce E. Dunn   (Eds.)

Telepathology

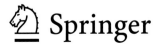

Springer

Sajeesh Kumar, Ph.D.
Department of Health Information Management
School of Health & Rehabilitation Sciences
University of Pittsburgh
6051 Forbes Tower
Pittsburgh, PA 15260, USA
sajeeshkr@yahoo.com

Bruce E. Dunn
Pathology and Laboratory Medicine Service (113)
Milwaukee Department of Veterans Affairs Hospital
5000 W. National Avenue
Milwaukee, WI 53295-1000, USA
Bruce.Dunn@va.gov

ISBN 978-3-540-85785-3   **e-ISBN 978-3-540-85786-0**
DOI: 10.1007/978-3-540-85786-0

Library of Congress Catalog Number: 2008934038

© Springer-Verlag Berlin Heidelberg 2009

Cover design: eStudio Calamar, Spain

Printed on acid-free paper

9 8 7 6 5 4 3 2 1

springer.com

Preface

Developments in telepathology are progressing at a great speed. As a consequence, there is a need for a broad overview of the field. This first ever book on telepathology is presented in such a way that it should make it accessible to anyone, independent of their knowledge of technology. The text is designed to be used by all professionals, including pathologists, surgeons, nurses and allied health professionals, and computer scientists.

In a very short time, driven by technical developments, the field of telepathology has become too extensive to be covered by only a small number of experts. Therefore, this Telepathology book has been written with chapter contributions from a host of renowned international authorities in telepathology (see the Table of Contents and the List of Contributors). This ensures that the subject matter focusing on recent advances in telepathology is truly up to date. Our guiding hope during this task was that as editors of multiple chapters we could still write with a single voice and keep the content coherent and simple. We hope that the clarity of this book makes up for any limitations in its comprehensiveness.

The editors took much care that this Telepathology book would not become merely a collection of separate chapters but, rather, would offer a consistent and structured overview of the field. We are aware that there is still considerable room for improvement and that certain elements of telepathology are not fully covered, such as legal and reimbursement policies. The editors invite readers, clinicians, and students to forward their valuable comments and feedback to further improve and expand future editions of this Telepathology book.

Books on theoretical and technical aspects inevitably use technical jargon, and this book is no exception. Although jargon is minimized, it cannot be eliminated without retreating to a more superficial level of coverage. The reader's understanding of the jargon will vary based on their backgrounds, but anyone with some background in computers, health, and/or biomedicine would be able to understand most of the terms used. In any case, an attempt to define all jargon terms has been made in the Glossary.

This Telepathology book has been organized systematically. The format and length of each chapter are standardized, thus ensuring that the content is concise and easy to read. Every chapter provides a comprehensive list of citations and references for further reading. Numerous figure drawings and clinical photographs throughout the book illustrate and illuminate the text well, providing its readers with high-quality visual reference material. Particularly useful features of this text are that each chapter has a summary of salient points for the reader.

The book consists of 16 chapters and begins with a brief introductory chapter explaining the basic concepts that are mainstay to telepathology, and subsequent chapters are built upon those foundations. Within each chapter, the goal is to provide a comprehensive overview of the topic. The final chapter covers future directions of telepathology.

This book would not have been possible without the contribution from various people. We acknowledge and appreciate the assistance of all reviewers and Ms. Latika Hans, editorial assistant from Bangalore, India. We thank all authors for making this book possible through their contributions and constant support.

SAJEESH KUMAR and BRUCE E. DUNN

Contents

Chapter 3
**Telepathology as an Essential Networking Tool
in VISN 12 of the United States Veterans**

BRUCE E. DUNN, HONGYUNG CHOI, DANIEL L. RECLA,
and THOMAS R. WISNIEWSKI

Chapter 4

GEORG HUTAREW

Chapter 5
Applications of Virtual Microscopy **53**
P.H.J. Riegman, W.N.M. Dinjens, M.H.A. Oomen,
W.F. Clotscher, R.J.J.R. Scholte, W. Sjoerdsma,
A.R.A. Riegman, and J.W. Oosterhuis

Chapter 9
Telepathology in Iran . . . .
AFSHIN ABDIRAD and SIAVASH GHADERI-SOHI

Chapter 10
Telepathology in Japan . . . .
TAKASHI SAWAI

Chapter 15
Remote Control of the Scanning Electron Microscope   205
ATSUSHI YAMADA

Chapter 16
Telepathology: An Audit.............................. **225**
Sᴀᴊᴇᴇsʜ Kᴜᴍᴀʀ

List of Contributors

Afshin Abdirad
Pathology Department, Cancer Institute of Tehran Medical University, Keshavarz Blvd., PO Box 14197-33141, Tehran, Iran
abdirada@sina.tums.ac.ir

Carlo A. Beltrami
Section of Pathology, Department of Medical and Morphological Research, University of Udine, Italy

Lajos Berczi
1st Department of Pathology and Experimental Oncology, Semmelweis University, VIII. Üllői út 26, 1085 Budapest, Hungary

Alexandra Maria Giovanna Brunasso
Department of Dermatology, Prato Hospital, Piazza dell' Ospedale, 59100 Prato, Italy
giovanna.brunasso@gmail.com

Klaus J. Busam
Weill Medical College of Cornell University, New York, NY, USA
Department of Pathology, Memorial Sloan–Kettering Cancer Center, 1275 York Avenue, New York, NY 10065, USA
busamk@mskcc.org

Palmina Cataldi
Azienda Sanitaria n.5, Palmanova, Italy

Hongyung Choi
Pathology and Laboratory Medicine Service (113), Clement J. Zablocki Veterans Affairs Medical Center, 5000 West National Avenue, Milwaukee, WI 53295-1000, USA
hongyung.choi@va.gov

W.F. Clotscher
Informatics Department, Erasmus MC, PO Box 2040,
3000 CA Rotterdam, The Netherlands

Mária Cserneky
1st Department of Pathology and Experimental Cancer Research,
Semmelweis University, VIII. Üllői út 26, 1085 Budapest, Hungary
mari@korb1.sote.hu

Vincenzo Della Mea
Medical Informatics, Telemedicine and eHealth Lab
Department of Mathematics and Computer Science
University of Udine, Via delle Scienze 206, 33100 Udine, Italy,
dellamea@dimi.uniud.it

Gionata De Vico
Dipartimento di Scienze Biologiche, Sezione di Zoologia,
Facoltà di Scienze MM.FF.NN.,
Università degli Studi di Napoli Federico II,
Via Mezzocannone 8, 80134 Napoli, Italy

W.N.M. Dinjens
Pathology Department, Erasmus MC, PO Box 2040
3000 CA Rotterdam, The Netherlands

Bruce E. Dunn
Pathology and Laboratory Medicine Service (113),
Milwaukee Department of Veterans Affairs Hospital
5000 W. National Avenue, Milwaukee, WI 53295-1000, USA
bruce.dunn@va.gov

Levente Ficsor
Digital Microscopy Laboratory, 2nd Department of Medicine,
Semmelweis University, VIII. Üllői út 26, 1085 Budapest, Hungary

László Fónyad
1st Department of Pathology and Experimental Cancer Research,
Semmelweis University, VIII. Üllői út 26, 1085 Budapest, Hungary
fonyadla@korb1.sote.hu

Siavash Ghaderi-Sohi
Pathology Department, Cancer Institute of Tehran Medical
University, Keshavarz Blvd., PO Box 14197-33141, Tehran, Iran

Georg Hutarew
Department of Pathology, Salzburg University Clinics (SALK)
Müllner Hauptstr. 48, 5020 Salzburg, Austria
g.hutarew@salk.at, hutarew@elsnet.at

Julie K. Karen
Clinical Assistant Professor of Dermatology
NYU School of Medicine, Laser & Skin Surgery of NY
317 East 34th Street, 11th Floor, New York, NY 10016, USA
jkkaren@gmail.com

Tibor Krenács
1st Department of Pathology and Experimental Cancer Research
Semmelweis University, VIII. Üllői út 26
1085 Budapest, Hungary
krenacst@korb1.sote.hu

Sajeesh Kumar
Department of Health Information Management
School of Health & Rehabilitation Sciences
University of Pittsburgh, 6051 Forbes Tower, Pittsburgh, PA 15260, USA
sajeeshkr@yahoo.com

Paola Maiolino
Dipartimento di Patologia e Sanità Animale,
Settore di Anatomia Patologica,
Facoltà di Medicina Veterinaria
Università degli Studi di Napoli Federico II
Via Delpino 1, 80137 Napoli, Italy
maiolino@unina.it

Cesare Massone
Research Unit of Teledermatology and Research Unit
of Dermatopathology, Department of Dermatology
Medical University of Graz, Auenbruggerplatz 8
8036 Graz, Austria
cesare.massone@klinikum-graz.at

Bela Molnar
Digital Microscopy Laboratory, 2nd Department of Medicine
Semmelweis University, VIII. Üllői út 26
1085 Budapest, Hungary
bela.molnar@3dhistech.com

Kishwer S. Nehal
Cornell Weill Medical College, New York, NY,
Memorial Sloan–Kettering Cancer Center, Dermatology Service
160 E. 53rd Street, 2nd Floor, New York, NY 10065, USA
nehalk@mskcc.org

M.H.A. Oomen
Pathology Department, Erasmus MC, PO Box 2040
3000 CA Rotterdam, The Netherlands

J.W. Oosterhuis
Pathology Department, Erasmus MC, PO Box 2040
3000 CA Rotterdam, The Netherlands

Barbara Pertoldi
Azienda Sanitaria, Palmanova, Italy

Aruna Prayaga
Professor of Pathology, Nizam's Institute of Medical Sciences
Punjagutta, Hyderabad 500 082, Andhra Pradesh, India
arunaprayaga56@yahoo.com

Daniel L. Recla
Pathology and Laboratory Medicine Service (113)
Iron Mountain Veterans Affairs Medical Center
325 East H Street, Iron Mountain, MI 49801, USA

A.R.A. Riegman
Pathology Department, Erasmus MC, PO Box 2040
3000 CA Rotterdam, The Netherlands

P.H.J. Riegman
Department of Pathology, Josephine Nefkens Institute Be 235b,
Erasmus Medical Center, Dr. Molewaterplein 40
3015 GG Rotterdam, The Netherlands
p.riegman@erasmusmc.nl

Takashi Sawai
Department of Pathology, School of Medicine
Iwate Medical University, 19-1 Uchimaru, Morioka
Iwate Prefecture 020-8505, Japan
tsawai@iwate-med.ac.jp

R.J.J.R. Scholte
Department of Education and Research, Erasmus MC
PO Box 2040, 3000 CA Rotterdam, The Netherlands

Josef A. Schroeder
Central EM-Lab, Pathology Department,
University Hospital Regensburg,
F.-J.-Strauss Allee 11, 93053 Regensburg, Germany
josef.schroeder@klinik.uni-regensburg.de

W. Sjoerdsma
Department of Education and Research, Erasmus MC
PO Box 2040, 3000 CA Rotterdam, The Netherlands

H. Peter Soyer
School of Medicine, Southern Clinical Division
The University of Queensland, Princess Alexandra Hospital
Brisbane QLD 4102, Australia
peter.soyer@telederm.eu, p.soyer@uq.edu.au

Béla Szende
1st Department of Pathology and Experimental Cancer Research
Semmelweis University, VIII. Üllői út 26
1085 Budapest, Hungary
bszende@korb1.sote.hu

Attila Tagscherer
3DHISTECH Ltd, Budapest, Hungary

Zsolt Tulassay
Digital Microscopy Laboratory, 2nd Department of Medicine,
VIII. Üllői út 26, 1085 Budapest, Hungary

Viktor Varga
Digital Microscopy Laboratory, 2nd Department of Medicine,
Semmelweis University, VIII. Üllői út 26
1085 Budapest, Hungary

Thomas R.Wisniewski
Pathology and Laboratory Medicine Service (113)
Clement J. Zablocki Veterans Affairs Medical Center
5000 West National Avenue,
Milwaukee WI 53295-1000, USA

Atsushi Yamada
Metrology Inspection Division SM Group
1-2 Musashino 3-Chome Akishima, Tokyo 196-8558, Japan
ayamada@jeol.co.jp

Abbreviations

AAPA	American Association of Pathologists' Assistants
AAV	Adeno(virus)-associated virus, used as a "ferry" in genetic molecular experiments
ACTS	Advanced communications technology and services
ADSL	Asymmetric digital subscriber line
AFIP	Armed Forces Institute of Pathology, Washington, DC, telediagnosis center
ASCUS	Atypical squamous cells of undetermined significance
ASP	Application service provider
ATI	American Telemedicine International
AVI	Audio video interleave
BCC	Basal cell carcinoma
BePro	Best practice in pathology and oncology
Bit	Unit of information in binary notation
BMP	BitMaP file format
BVCS	Bitfield video communication system
CADASIL	Cerebral autosomal-dominant artheriopathy with subcortical infarcts and leukoencephalopathy
CCD	Charge-coupled device
cDNA	Complementary DNA (or spliced DNA) synthesized using a special enzyme and used in genetic molecular techniques
CEN	Central European country
CI	Confidence interval
COMPO	Backscattered composition electron image
CON	Consensus diagnosis
CPC	Clinicopathological conference
CPU	Central processing unit
CT	Computed tomography
DICOM	Digital imaging and communications in medicine

DNA	Deoxyribonucleic acid
DPI	Dots per inch
EELS	Electron energy loss spectroscopy
EFTEM	Energy-filtered transmission electron microscope
EM	Electron microscopy/microscope
EORTC	European Organisation for Research and Treatment of Cancer
EQA	External quality assessment/external quality assurance
ESI	Electron spectroscopic imaging
EU	European Union
EUS	Endoscopic ultrasound
FCIF	Full common intermediate format
FISH	Fluorescence in situ hybridization
FNA	Fine-needle aspiration
FOV	Field of view
Fps	Frames (images) per second
FTP	File transfer protocol
FTTH	Fiber to the home
GB	Gigabyte(s)
GDS	Global dialing scheme
GHz	Gigahertz
H&E	Hematoxylin and eosin
HBONE	Hungarian Backbone Network
HDSF	Hybrid, dynamic store and forward
HPV	Human papillomavirus
HTML	Hypertext markup language
IAP	International Academy of Pathology
ICT	Information and communication technologies
ID	Identification
IHC	Immunohistochemistry
IIF	Information Infrastructure Development
INSERM	Institut National de la Sante et de la Recherche Medicale, Nantes, France
IP	Internet protocol
iPATH Basel	Verein zur Förderung der Telemedizin, telediagnosis server located in Basel, Switzerland
ISDN	Integrated Services Digital Network
ISRO	Indian Space Research Organisation
IT	Information technology
JEOL	Japan Electron Optics Laboratory

JPEG	Computer format for compressing images (Joint Photographic Experts Group)
JPEG2000	Image compression standard
JRST–TI	Japanese Research Society of Telepathology and Telepathology Informatics
JRST–VM	Japanese Research Society of Telepathology–Virtual Microscopy
JSP	Japanese Society of Pathology
$1\,k \times 1\,k$	$1{,}024 \times 1{,}024$ (pixels)
kV	1,000 V
LAN	Local area network
LEO	Now called ZEISS, electron microscopy manufacturer
mm	1/1,000,000 m
Mbps	Megabit per second
MB RAM	Megabite random access memory
MCU	Multipoint control unit
MHz	1,000,000 Hz
MIA	Multiple image alignment
MLHW	Ministry of Health, Labor, and Welfare
MMA	Miniaturized microscope array
MMC	Materials Microcharacterization Collaboratory, ORNL, USA
MSA	Microscopy Society of America
msec	Millisecond
MSKCC	Memorial Sloan–Kettering Cancer Center
MV	1,000,000 V
NCMIR	National Center for Microscopy and Imaging Research, San Diego, USA
NFD/NSF	Nephrogenic Fibrosing Dermopathy/Nephrogenic Systemic Fibrosis
NIIF	National Information Infrastructure Development Institute
NIL	Negative for intraepithelial lesion
nm	1/1,000,000,000 m
OB/GYN	Obstetrician/gynecologist
OECI	Organisation of European Cancer Institutes
OM	Optical microscope
ORNL/TE	Oak Ridge National Laboratory, Tennessee, USA
OS	Operating system
OSIS	Olympus Soft Imaging Systems GmbH, Muenster, Germany

PACS	Picture archival and communication system
PAS	Periodic acid-Schiff
PC	Personal computer
PCMCIA	Personal Computer Memory Card International Association, computer device
PCR	Polymerase chain reaction
PET-scan	Positron emission tomography scan
POP	Point of presence
PRAGMA	Pacific Rim and Grid Middleware Assembly
RAM	Random axis memory
RPE65	A human gene encoding the retinal pigment epithelium-specific protein 65 Da
SACS	Slide archive and communication system
SAF	Store and forward
SARS	Severe acute respiratory syndrome
SCC	Squamous cell carcinoma
SCUR	Society for Cutaneous Ultrastructure Research
SEI	Secondary electron image
SEM	Scanning electron microscope
SIS	Now OSIS, Olympus Soft Imaging System GmbH, Muenster, Germany
SNOMED	Systematized nomenclature of medicine
TCP/IP	Transmission control protocol/internet protocol
TEM	Transmission electron microscope
TFT	Thin-film transistor, used in flat screen monitors
TIFF	Tagged image file format
TMA	Tissue microarray
TOPO	Backscattered topography electron image
TRS	Manufacturer of digital cameras for electron microscopes, Moorenweis, Germany
UICC Berlin	Union Internationale Contre Le Cancer, telediagnosis center located at Charité in Berlin, Germany
UMTS	Universal Mobile Telecommunications System, third generation of cell phone technology
USB	Universal serial bus
VAMC	Veterans Affairs Medical Center
VATS	Video-assisted thoracoscopic surgery
VHA	United States Veterans Health Administration
VISN	Veterans Integrated Service Networks
VM	Virtual microscope
VPN	Virtual Private Network

VS	Virtual slide
VSS	Virtual slide system
WAN	Wide area network
WEB-SEM	Web-based scanning electron microscope
WLAN	Wireless local area network
WSI	Whole slide imaging
WWM Japan	World Wide Microscope, telediagnosis system from Japan
XML	Extensible markup language
YAG	Yttrium aluminum garnet, a scintillator used in CCD cameras

Introduction to Telepathology

Sajeesh Kumar

1.1
Introduction to Telemedicine

Telemedicine is a method by which patients can be examined, investigated, monitored, and treated, with the patient and the doctor being located at different places. Tele is a Greek word meaning "distance," and Mederi is a Latin word meaning, "to heal." Although initially considered "futuristic" and "experimental," telemedicine is today a reality and has come to stay. In telemedicine, one transfers the expertise, not the patient. Hospitals of the future will drain patients from all over the world without geographical limitations. High-quality medical services can be brought to the patient, rather than transporting the patient to distant and expensive tertiary-care centers. A major goal of telemedicine is to eliminate unnecessary traveling of patients and their escorts. Image acquisition, image storage, image display and processing, and image transfer represent the basis of telemedicine. Telemedicine is becoming an integral part of health-care services in several countries.

1.2
What Is Telepathology?

Telepathology is a branch of telemedicine and pathology that use telecommunication technology to facilitate the transfer of image-rich pathology data between remote locations for the purposes of diagnosis, education, and research. Typically, this is done over standard telephone lines, wide area network (WAN), or a local area network (LAN). Through telepathology, images can be sent to another part of the hospital, or to other locations around the world.

Telepathology systems are divided into three major types: static image-based systems, real-time systems, and virtual slide systems. Static image systems have major benefits of being the most reasonably priced and most usable in the widest range of settings but have the significant drawback in only being able to capture a selected subset of microscopic fields. Real-time systems and virtual slides allow a consultant pathologist the opportunity to evaluate the entire specimen. With real-time systems, the consultant actively operates a microscope located at a distant site – changing focus, illumination, magnification, and field of view at will. Virtual slide systems use an automated scanner that takes a visual image of the entire slide, which can then be forwarded to another location for diagnosis.

While real-time and virtual slide systems appear ideal for telepathology, there are certain drawbacks to each. Real-time systems perform best on LANs, but performance may suffer if employed during periods of high network traffic or using the Internet proper as a backbone. The scanning of virtual slides, at this point, is still a time-intensive operation, requiring anywhere from minutes to hours to accurately scan a single slide. Expense is also an issue with real-time and virtual slide systems, as they can be costly.

1.3
Scope of Telepathology

The use of telepathology is of great importance in management of patients, since it allows fast diagnosis and interconsultations among specialist pathologists located in any part of the world.

Telepathology, which is the diagnostic work of a pathologist at a distance, has been developed to routine application. It can be classified in relation to application, technical solutions, or performance conditions. Diagnostic pathology performance distinguishes primary diagnosis (e.g., frozen section statement) from secondary diagnosis (e.g., expert consultation) and quality assurance (diagnostic accuracy, continuous education, and training). Applications comprise (1) frozen section service, (2) expert consultations, (3) remote control measurements, and (4) education and training.

The technical solutions distinguish active (remote control, live imaging) systems from passive (conventional microscope handling, static imaging), and the performance systems with interactive (online, live imaging) use from those with passive (offline, static imaging) practice. Intraoperative frozen section service is mainly performed with remote control systems, whereas expert consultations and education/training are commonly based on Internet connections with static imaging in an offline mode. The image quality, transfer rates, and screen resolution of active and passive telepathology systems are sufficient for an additional or primary judgment of histological slides and cytological smears.

From the technical point of view, remote control telepathology requires a fast transfer and at least near online judgment of images, i.e., image acquisition, transfer, and presentation can be considered one performance function. Thus, image size, line transfer rate, and screen resolution define the practicability of the system. In expert consultation, the pixel resolution of images and natural color presentation are the main factors for diagnostic support, whereas the line transfer rate is of minor importance. These conditions define the technical compartments, especially size and resolution of camera and screen. The performance of commercially available systems has reached a high-quality standard. Pathologists can be trained in a short time and can use the systems in a routine manner. Several telepathology systems have been implemented in large institutes of pathology, which serve for frozen section diagnosis in small hospitals located in the local area. In contrast, expert consultation is mainly performed with international connections.

In expansion of these experiences, a "globalization" of telepathology can be expected. Telepathology can be used to shrink the period necessary for final diagnosis by requesting diagnostic assistance from colleagues working in appropriate related time zones. Telepathology is, therefore, not a substitute of conventional diagnostic procedures, but a real improvement in the world of pathology.

Potential applications of telepathology may also include:

- Training new pathologists
- Assisting and training pathologists in developing countries
- Diagnose injured soldiers on or near the battlefield
- Performing pathological procedures in space
- Collaborating and mentoring by pathologists around the globe

1.4
Relevance of Telepathology in Developing Countries

Ideally, every citizen in the world should have immediate access to the appropriate specialist for medical consultation. However, the current status of the health service is such that total medical care cannot be provided in rural areas. Even secondary and tertiary medical care is not uniformly available in suburban and urban areas. Incentives to entice specialist pathologists to practice in suburban or rural areas have failed in many nations.

It is generally considered that the communities most likely to benefit from *telepathology* are those least likely to afford it or to have the requisite communication infrastructure. However, this may no longer be true. In contrast to the bleak scenario in health care, Internet connections and computer literacy are fast developing, and prices are falling. Theoretically, it is far easier to set up an excellent telecommunication infrastructure in suburban and rural areas than to place hundreds of medical specialists in these places. The world has realized that the future of telecommunications lies in satellite-based technology and fiber-optic cables. Providing health care in remote areas using high technology is not as absurd as it may initially appear. Could even the greatest optimist have anticipated the phenomenal explosion in the use of computers in the villages of India?

1.5
Summary

- Telemedicine aids in examination, investigation, monitoring, and treatment of patients who are located away from the physician.
- Telepathology is a branch of telemedicine and pathology that use telecommunication technology to facilitate the transfer of image-rich pathology data between remote locations.
- A telepathology system can be divided into three major types: static image-based systems, real-time systems, and virtual slide systems.
- Telepathology is of great importance in management of patients, since it allows fast diagnosis and interconsultations among specialist pathologists located at different places.

Digital Slide and Virtual Microscopy-Based Routine and Telepathology Evaluation of Gastrointestinal Biopsy Specimen

Bela Molnar, Lajos Berczi, Levente Ficsor, Viktor Varga, Attila Tagscherer, and Zsolt Tulassay

2.1
Introduction

Medical digital image analysis, following the rapid developments in the information technology industry, is getting more and more an accepted method [21]. Digital techniques and laboratories [7] already exist for the radiology applications. New standalone automated microscope systems and recently fully automated digital slide scanners were developed for the histo/cytology applications in the last decade and years as well.

The automated rescreening of cervical smears is now available for routine [14, 17]. Several new semiautomatic microscopes were developed for the quality control of the cytotechnologists' work [1, 2, 12, 13]. These systems notify the scanned area and images, and additional electronic recording of selected images is also available. The automated histological analysis is important research project for several years, but the results were unsatisfactory for routine applications [3, 19]. However, the histological diagnosis can be supported already today by new electronic techniques like the TV image cytometry and teleconsultation based on histological images rather than entire samples [6].

Telepathology services were built in the last decade around two technology platforms. The dynamic telepathology includes remote-controlled microscope systems with high-throughput online image transport channels [8, 27]. This method has the advantage of entire slide access and lacks the error source of preselected microscopic frames; however, the costs of the system and working are relatively high. The application of static preselected images for teleconsultation needs much less hardware investment; however, a sampling error can occur [25, 26]. Using Internet as a telecommunication pathway for static images is a low-cost widely available alternative [9, 11].

The application of a digital slide should be considerable as a source and target of the telepathology and automated histological analysis. In the last years, attempts to use an electronic or digital slide for education, teleconsultation, and immunohistochemical analysis are growing [4, 5, 15, 23]. The storage capacity and speed of personal computers became applicable only recently for handling the huge amount of image information stored on a slide.

Low-cost, commercial, motorized microscopes were marketed by several manufacturers in late 1990s. Recently, several automated digital slide scanning systems became widely available and used for transmitted light and multichannel fluorescence. They are using either optical elements of the microscopy with a CCD camera or a line sensor. A special alternative could be the multilens slide scanning systems.

Working on digital slides should require virtual or digital microscopy. Preliminary positive results on a limited number of mosaicked microscopic images have been reported recently [22].

The aim of the study was the evaluation of a digital slide scanning system and a virtual microscope (VM) on gastrointestinal biopsy specimen in a routine environment. A comparison was performed between the optical microscope (OM) and digital microscope evaluation in local and remote mode.

2.2
Materials and Methods

2.2.1
Gastric Routine Biopsy Specimen Analysis

Biopsy specimens were placed in buffered formalin, routinely processed and stained with hematoxylin and eosin. Altogether 103 specimens were selected from the files of cases seen at the Ist Department of Pathology. Single representative slide was evaluated from each case. The distribution of the cases is listed in Table 2.1.

The histological sections were evaluated in separate setting on the VM and OM without the knowledge of the previous analysis by two independent, board-certified histologists. First, the evaluation of the glass slides on optical microscopy was done. The paper copies of the clinical histories and the evaluation report were collected. In several weeks, the slides were digitized by our system described in later sections by an assistant.

The slide digitization was done in the Digital Microscopy Laboratory. The scanning computer was used as a digital slide server too. The virtual microscopy evaluation was done on a separate local area network (LAN) workstation in the

Table 2.1. Diagnoses

Organ	Diagnoses	No. of cases
Gastric	Healthy	5
	Chronic gastritis without intestinal metaplasia	16
	Chronic gastritis with intestinal metaplasia	12
	Chronic gastritis with atrophia	3
	Adenocarcinoma well differentiated, intestinal type	9
	Adenocarcinoma, nondifferentiated	6
	Sigillocellular carcinoma	4
	Anaplastic carcinoma	2
	Adenopapillar carcinoma	1
	Hyperplastic polyp	1
	MALT lymphoma	2
Colon	Healthy	5
	Colitis ulcerosa	14
	Crohn's disease	7
	Chr. Asp. colitis	4
	Hyperplastic polyp	2
	Adenoma tubulare with severe dysplasia	2
	Adenoma tubulovillosum with severe dysplasia	1
	Adenoma papillare	1
	Adenoma tubulopapillare	1
	Adenoma villosum with dysplasia	1
	Adenocarcinoma	4

Pathology Department with access to the slide server computer using the Internet (Fig. 2.1).

2.2.2
Data Analysis

At the conclusion of the study, having all the optical and virtual microscopy results and the consensus data, concordance and source of diagnostic discordance were determined.

Concordance was designated level "a." Levels "b" and "c" were either clinically unimportant or clinically important discordance, as suggested by Weinberg et al. [25].

The cases where discordant results were observed were collected together with the optical and electronic data. The final diagnosis and definition of the source of the discordant data were brought by consensus diagnosis (CON) on a common session in the consultation room. Here, the access to the digital slides was also available through a computer workstation and Internet.

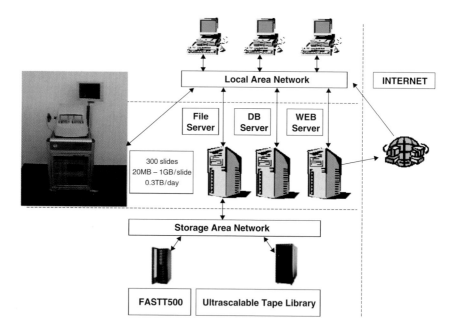

Fig. 2.1. Databank behind the Mirax digital slides. Slides can be stored on the scanning PC, on a dedicated slide server, dispatched through the Web directly. Slide images and patient information can be stored separately. Long-term storage application is included on tape libraries

The reasons for discordance were classified by the consensus meeting as to inadequate image quality (class I), interpretation (class II), and insufficient clinical information (class III). The significance of the concordance was determined using Kendall's concordance coefficient determined by the Statistica program package (V.4.3, Statsoft, USA).

2.2.3
Slide Digitization and the VM System

2.2.3.1
Used Hardware Tools

We used a Mirax Scan digital slide scanner (developed and produced by 3DHISTECH Ltd, Budapest; distributed worldwide by Carl Zeiss, Jena, Germany) (Fig. 2.2). This scanner allows the fully automated scanning of up to 300 slides in a batch, using slide magazines each for 50 slides. The automated identification of the slides is done through the barcode label. Automated identification of area of interest is done through a preview camera. The microscope functions (objectives, stage, focus, illumination, and filters) can be controlled and changed

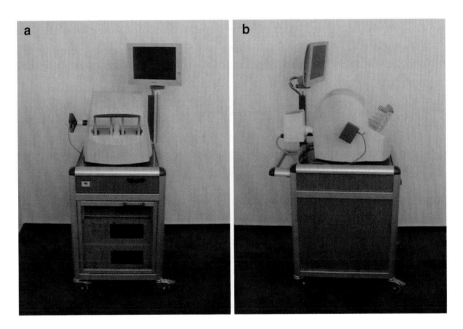

Fig. 2.2. The Mirax scanner developed for high-throughput automated scanning of large-volume slides. (**a**) Frontal view with the stage and control computers. (**b**) Side view: view of the camera, fluorescent illumination. Note the slide magazines on the loading rack

through the RS232 interface from an application program. The mechanic accuracy of the motorized scanning stage for X/Y and Z directions was 0.3 µm.

In our work, we used the Allied Vision Technologies Marlin 1,4 MP one-chip CCD camera with 1,380 × 1,030 pixels. The integration time of the camera can be controlled through the computer interface RS485. The programs were running on computers with a double-core Intel processor, 128 MB RAM, and 2 GB hard disk. The scanning time for a biopsy, including loading, barcode identification, scanning, and slide repositioning into the slide holding magazine, is between 2 and 4 min.

2.2.3.2
Features of the Digital Slide Scanning Program

1. Calibration of the microscope, scanning stage, camera resolution.
2. Slide loading.
3. Barcode reading and identification.
4. Scanning area determination after preview scanning.
5. Autoscanning was started after setting the stage at zero position. In the scanning process, autofocusing was done only at each 3–5 field of view. Each of the images was compressed in JPEG and stored in the slide databank in the corresponding position. Autofocusing was done using Brenner's algorithm [10]. At 40× objective, 125,856 frames would have to be stored for the entire slide. However, a threshold filter was used to store only frames with image content. This way only the area of a biopsy was stored, which means 160–700 frames per slide.
6. First, the mosaicking of the field of views was done using mathematical algorithms [20]; however, the error of the stage between the required and real position was proved to be less than +0.5 µm. A high-precision software mosaicking alignment was used for stitching of the single field of views (Fig. 2.3).

2.2.3.3
Features of the VM Program

1. *Slide selection.* After scanning, the slides are stored in subdirectories called *projects* for a higher ordering. After selection, an electronically minimized slide image is shown on the screen (Fig. 2.4).
2. *Slide orientation maps.* This map represents the whole slide, where one pixel on the screen corresponds to one field of view. The recorded segments are labeled with white pixels on a gray background.

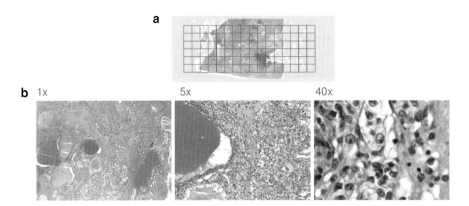

Fig. 2.3. (**a**) Scanning principle of the Mirax system: the sample on the slide is recorded in stitched mosaic of single field of views. (**b**) Digital magnification of a digital slide

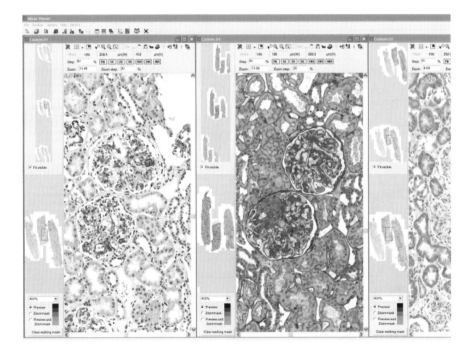

Fig. 2.4. User interface of the MIRAX viewer software. Image of the slide, intermedier magnification of the slide, and virtual microscopy are available for perfect orientation. Parallel viewing of the same specimen is available with different sections and staining in oriented and multiple windows

3. *Applicable electronic magnifications.* After finding the interested area, the user has several options for magnification of the selected segments. One can use the prepared magnification steps of 100× and 200× or special "+" and "−" mouse arrows to change the magnification.

4. *Moving and scrolling the slide.* If the interested area is not on the screen in the required magnification on the slide, then the moving arrows (up, down, left, and right) can be used to move the slide into any directions.

5. *Labelling of interested frames for re-evaluation, consultation, and reporting.* Up to ten colored labels can be placed on the digital slide in the software. This option can also be used for reconsultation by experts via LAN or in specific cases via Internet.

6. *Internet access.* The scanning computer can be used as a slide server too. However, uploading to a central digital slide repository with safety options can be performed automatically. We used the PATHONET portal for digital slide storing and dispatch through the Internet (http://www.pathonet.com) (Fig. 2.5). This way homework and consultation became easily available.

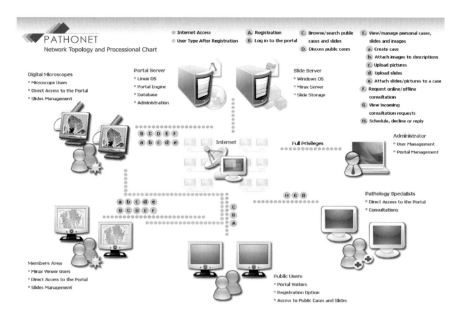

Fig. 2.5. Concept and functions of the PATHONET portal (http://www.pathonet.com) for users with scanner or viewer. Active (up- and download of slides) and passive (viewing, library access) usages are available. Parallel viewing for closed participant network is available with options for publication-related digital slide handling, quality-control networks, and education applications

In the case of direct access to the slide server, the slide server's IP address has to be defined on the remote workstation. After connecting to the server computer, the list of the available slides and their information is transported to the client workstation. After selecting a slide, its electronically compressed low-resolution image is transferred to the workstation. Every image that is transported during the evaluation will be stored on the local machine for safety reasons.

2.3
Results

2.3.1
Concordance

In altogether seven cases (6.7%), discordance was found between VM or OM and the CON. In four cases the OM and in three cases the VM yielded the correct diagnosis.

Out of the 103 cases, in 96 (93.2%) concordance and in 98 (95.1%) clinically important concordance were found. OM yielded similar (100/103, 97%) concordance with the consensus results than the VM (99/103, 96.1%). For the clinically important diagnosis, a similar concordance was also observed (Table 2.2).

2.3.2
Reasons for Diagnostic Discordance

In our study due to the fact that the entire specimen was digitized, we could not have sampling error. However, the other common sources of errors in telepathology, interpretation (4/7), or insufficient clinical information (3/7)

Table 2.2. Concordance between optical microscopy, virtual microscopy, and the consensus diagnosis

	Concordance all types (%)	Concordance clinically important (%)
OM vs. VM	93.2 (96/103)	95.1 (98/103)
OM vs. Con	97.0 (100/103)	98.0 (101/103)
VM vs. Con	96.1 (98/103)	97.1 (100/103)

OM optical microscope, *VM* virtual microscope, *Con* consensus

Table 2.3. Reasons of diagnostic discordance

Level discordance	Reason of discordance	VM diagnoses	Optical micro-scopy diagnosis	Review consensus diagnosis
B	II	Chronic gastritis	Acute and chronic gastritis	VM
C	III	Gastric adenoma	Gastric hyper-plastic polyp	VM
C	II	Chronic atrophic gastritis	Chronic gastritis with low-grade dysplasia	OM
B	II	Hyperplastic polyp	Hyperplastic mucosa	OM
C	II	Mild colitis	Normal colon	OM
C	III	Colitis ulcerosa with dysplasia	Colitis ulcerosa	VM
C	III	Adenoma papillare	Hyperplastic polyp	OM

Discordance: *B* clinically not important, *C* clinically important
Reason of discordance: *I* image quality, *II* interpretation, *III* insufficient clinical information

could be observed (Table 2.3). With the advances in optical imaging (higher-resolution, multiple focus levels), no image quality errors were found.

2.3.3
Technical and Practical Data at the Application of VM

The hard-disk volume of a microscopic field of view is between 60 and 100 KB after JPEG compression. The overall hard-disk place for a gastric biopsy is between 30 and 50 MB, and the scanning time is between 20 and 40 min, depending on the number and area of sections on a slide. The evaluation of the specimen on the monitor is more comfortable and more reproducible and docu-mentable, as compared to the optical way (Table 2.4).

In the Internet remote access, the speed of the transfer was relatively fast. The first minimized image was uploaded in the real time. As the user switched over

Table 2.4. Comparison between optical and virtual microscope evaluation methods

Microscopy feature	Optical evaluation	Electronic evaluation
Speed	4–5 min	2–3 min
Costs	Every user, high-quality microscope	One high-quality scanning microscope
		Image server
		Evaluation terminal
Working conditions	Only limited number of slides can be evaluated because of fatigue	Normal monitor work
Consultation	With slide transportation or with image transfer through ISDN, telephone line, and Internet	Remote access to the image server through LAN or Internet
Quality control	With special additional hardware	By recording of evaluated image segments

to high magnification, the single field of views was demonstrated on the screen in seconds. The application of portal technology allowed the parallel viewing of the slides in different geographical locations, yielding CON opportunities through the Web.

2.4
Discussion

In this work, the technical feasibility and user acceptance of a digital histological section evaluation system were shown. Using high-end automated digital slide scanners, advanced PC technology, now a real-life application of digital histology, became available.

These developments and results prove that in the near future, we can have microscope-free virtual microscopy workstations with the function of the OM. On one side, it would mean more working comfort for the histologists. On the other side, it would also support quality-control techniques and consultation with remote experts as well. The primary application of digital slides and virtual microscopy should be now the routine sign-out and not only the consultation.

Remote evaluation of the slides through Internet includes the advantages of the previously used static or dynamic telepathology methods (entire slide is available in high magnification, microscope, and remote assistance-free evaluation) [24].

The observed concordance with optical microscopy was higher than in previous static image-based telepathology studies [25–27]. This can be explained by the fact that this technology eliminates the sampling error. Evaluation of certainty, time constraints, and fatigue was not done. It is considered to be done in a larger interlaboratory study.

The digitization of the routine specimen for Intranet or telediagnostics could be performed directly in the H/E sample preparation laboratory. The Mirax scanner has slide magazines with 50 slides each. In the routine workflow in the biopsy laboratory, the coverslipping is done also in batches of 50–60 slides. In our laboratory, the first set of H/E-stained, coverslipped slides are ready at 11:00 a.m. Using the high-speed scanning, the first set of slides are on the workstations monitor at between 11:20 and 11:30. The routine sign-out can happen directly, and an electronic report could be prepared on the monitor and sent out even in an email in seconds.

O'Brien and Sotnikov [18] defined in their 1996 review article about the computerization of the histology laboratory as a desirable but far future. Leong and McGee [16] published recently that automated complete slide digitization has influence on all levels of the clinical practice and education. They emphasized the importance of a dedicated software technology for the practical use.

The results of our study showed that the digital slide and virtual microscopy technology can be used in selected cases for telepathology consultation, but not for everyday routine use.

2.5
Summary

- Automated digital slide scanning became available in the last years through digital slide scanners.
- Their pilot application on gastrointestinal specimen is rational due to the volume of the biopsy sections.
- Teleconsultation through Intra- and Internet are both applicable alternatives.
- The concordance between optical and virtual microscopy results to concordance diagnosis is similarly high due to image quality developments in the digital slide scanning technology.

■ The application of virtual microscopy with digital slide scanners for gastro-intestinal biopsy specimen telepathology is now supported by the results of our study.

References

1. Anderson TL, Nelson AC (1995) Quality control and proficiency testing of cytological smear screening: an integrated approach using automation. In: Wied GL, Keebler CM, Rosenthal DL, Schenck U, Somrak TM, Vooijs GP (eds) Compendium on quality assurance, proficiency testing and workload limitations on clinical cytology. Tutorials of Cytology, Chicago, IL, pp. 83–287
2. Baker RW, Wadsworth J, Brugal G, Coleman DV (1998) An evaluation of 'rapid review' as a method of quality control of cervical smears using the AxioHOME microscope. Cytopathology 8:85–95
3. Belhomme P, Elmoataz A, Herlin P, Bloyet D (1996) Generalised region growing operator with optimal scanning: application to segmentation of breast cancer images. J Microsc 886:41–50
4. Burns BF (1997) Creating low power photomicrographs using a 35 mm digital slide scanner. Am J Surg Pathol 21:865–866
5. Dee FR (2006) Virtual microscopy for comparative pathology. Toxicol Pathol 34:966–973
6. Dictor M (1997) The surgical pathologist in a client/server computer network: work support, quality assurance, and the graphical user interface. Mod Pathol 10:259–266
7. Dooley RL, Engel C, Muller ME (1997) Automated scanning and digitizing of roentgenographs for documentation and research. Clin Orthop 274:113–119
8. Dunn BE, Almagro UA, Choi H, et al (1997) Dynamic-robotic telepathology: department of Veteran Affairs feasibility. Hum Pathol 28:8–12
9. Eusebi V, Foschini L, Erde S, et al (1997) Transcontinental consults in surgical pathology via the Internet. Hum Pathol 28:13–16
10. Firestone L, Cook K, Culp K (1991) Comparison of autofocus methods for automated microscopy. Cytometry 12:195–206
11. Gombas P, Szende B, Stotz G (1996) Support by telecommunications in diagnostic pathology. Experience with the first telepathology system in Hungary. Orv Hetilap 137:2299–2303
12. Grohs DH, Gombrich PP, Domanik RA (1996) AccuMed International, Inc. Meeting the challenges in cervical cancer screening: the AcCell Series 2000 automated slide handling and data management system. Acta Cytol 40:26–30
13. Grohs DH, Dadeshidze VV, Domanik RA, Gombrich PP, Olsson LJ, Pressman NJ (1997) Utility of the TracCell system in mapping *Papanicolaou*-stained cytologic material. Acta Cytol 41:144–152
14. Hailey DM, Lea R (1995) Prospects for newer technologies in cervical cancer screening programmes. J Qual Clin Pract 15:139–145
15. Helin HO, Lundin ME, Laakso M, Lundin J, Helin HJ, Isola J (2006) Virtual microscopy in prostate histopathology: simultaneous viewing of biopsies stained sequentially with hematoxylin and eosin, and alpha-methylacyl-coenzyme A racemase/p63 immunohistochemistry. J Urol 175:459–504
16. Leong FJWM, McGee O'D (2001) Automated complete slide digitization: a medium for simultaneous viewing by multiple pathologists. J Pathol 195:508–514

17. Mango LJ, Ivasauskas EZ (1995) Computer assisted cervical cytology using the PAPNET testing. In: Wied GL, Keebler CM, Rosenthal DL, Schenck U, Somrak TM, Vooijs GP (eds) Compendium on quality assurance, proficiency testing and workload limitations on clinical cytology. Tutorials of Cytology, Chicago, IL, pp. 155–167

18. O'Brien MJ, Sotnikov AV (1996) Digital imaging in anatomic pathology. Am J Clin Pathol 106:25–32

19. Ong SH, Jin XC, Sinniah R (1996) Image analysis of tissue sections. Comput Biol Med 26:269–279

20. Ott SR (1997) Acquisition of high-resolution digital images in video microscopy: automated image mosaicking on a desktop microcomputer. Microsc Res Tech 38:335–343

21. Shotton DM (1995) Robert Feulgen Prize Lecture 1995. Electronic light microscopy: present capabilities and future prospects. Histochem Cell Biol 104:97–137

22. Singson RPC, Natarajan S, Greenson JK, Marchevsky AM (1999) Virtual microscopy and the Internet as telepathology consultation tools. A study of gastrointestinal biopsy specimens. Am J Pathol 111:792–795

23. Stewart J III, Myazaki K, Bevans-Wilkins K (2007) Virtual microscopy for cytology proficiency testing: are we there yet? Cancer 111:203–212

24. Weinberg DS (1996) How is telepathology being used to improve patient care. Clin Chem 42:831–835

25. Weinberg DS, Allaert FA, Dusserre P, et al (1996) Telepathology diagnosis by means of digital still images: an international validation study. Hum Pathol 27:111–118

26. Weinstein RS (1996) Prospects for telepathology. Hum Pathol 17:433–434

27. Weinstein RS, Battacharayya AK, Graham AR, et al (1997) Telepathology a ten-year progress report. Hum Pathol 28:1–7

Telepathology as an Essential Networking Tool in VISN 12 of the United States Veterans Health Administration

Bruce E. Dunn, Hongyung Choi, Daniel L. Recla, and Thomas R. Wisniewski

3.1
Background

Telepathology involves the sending and viewing of video and digitized images for the purpose of rendering primary or consultative diagnoses by pathologists at a distance [13, 15, 23, 24]. This technology has facilitated reorganization of the Veterans Health Administration (VHA) pathology labs in several regions of the United States. Starting in 1995, the VHA has reorganized into 21 Veterans Integrated Service Networks (VISNs). The seven Veterans Affairs Medical Centers (VAMCs) currently comprising VISN 12 are located in a roughly rectangular geographic region, measuring approximately 320 miles in north–south direction and 100 miles in east–west direction in the Upper Midwest. Lake Michigan forms the eastern geographic border for much of VISN 12. The VAMCs include Iron Mountain, MI; Tomah, WI; Madison, WI; Milwaukee, WI; North Chicago, IL; Hines, Maywood, IL (suburban Chicago); and Chicago, IL. Figure 3.1 shows the distances in miles between the VAMCs from Milwaukee, which is centrally located. The Iron Mountain and Tomah VAMCs are rural, are not affiliated with medical schools, and have no on-site pathologist. The North Chicago VAMC is affiliated with a medical school but does not have an on-site pathologist. The remaining four VAMCs are affiliated with medical schools and have on-site pathologists. Since 2005, the North Chicago VAMC has been actively engaged in consolidation with the former Great Lakes Naval Hospital (now Clinic), operated by the Department of the Navy. Complete consolidation of clinical services is scheduled to occur by 2010. The Tomah VAMC does not maintain an inpatient surgery program, whereas the other six medical centers support inpatient surgery.

In mid-1996, we implemented a routine surgical telepathology service using a commercially available, robotic, hybrid dynamic store-and-forward (HDSF) telepathology system between the Iron Mountain and Milwaukee VAMCs

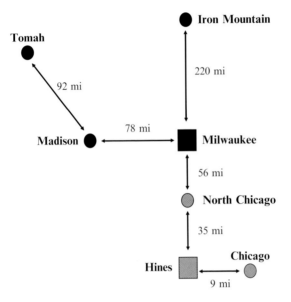

Fig. 3.1. Relative locations and distances between the seven Veterans Affairs Medical Centers located within Veterans Integrated Service Network 12. Distances are shown in miles (mi). Iron Mountain is the northernmost medical center, while Hines and Chicago are the southernmost medical centers in VISN 12. Tomah and Madison are located on the west side of the network. Lake Michigan (not shown) forms the eastern border for most of VISN 12. The medical centers in *black* form the northern tier of VISN 12, for which Milwaukee (*square*) serves as the core laboratory. The medical centers shown in *gray* form the southern tier of VISN 12, for which Hines (*square*) serves as the core laboratory

[8, 9, 11, 12]. Using robotic telepathology, a pathologist located at a distance from the actual microscope is able to control slide movement, as well as select and control magnification, focus, and lighting [11, 12]. Live (dynamic) and static (still) images are viewed in real time on a computer screen. The rationale for implementing telepathology was that upon retirement of the former part-time, on-site pathologist, the chief of staff at Iron Mountain requested that Milwaukee provide services by telepathology. Among the perceived advantages of telepathology were the ability to access multiple medical school-affiliated pathologists, the provision of uninterrupted service in the case of an absence of a given pathologist, and the ability to streamline the reporting process.

At about the same time that telepathology was initially implemented between Iron Mountain and Milwaukee, reorganization of services and greater emphasis on cost effectiveness lead to the creation of a consolidated pathology and laboratory service line in VISN 12. The impetus for development of the consolidated service line was improved efficiency through reduction of employees (by attrition) and decreased service redundancy. Within the service line, laboratories at Hines and Milwaukee were designated as core (hub) laboratories, while those at the remaining sites were designated as primary (remote) laboratories.

Starting in 1998, based on the positive telepathology experiences between Iron Mountain and Milwaukee VAMCs, VISN 12 chose to achieve real-time connectivity between the eight then-existent VAMC hospital-based laboratories, to provide a single standard of accurate, timely pathology service. Subsequently, two of the medical centers (Lakeside and West Side) merged to form the Chicago (Jesse Brown) VAMC. The available equipment selected (Apollo Telemedicine, Falls Church, VA) included the only commercial robotic telepathology system available at the time. Each VISN 12 laboratory has a single telepathology workstation linked to a private wide area network (WAN). The WAN has been described previously [13, 14]. The telepathology system uses a combination of nonrobotic and robotic HDSF telepathology systems (Fig. 3.2). The only robotic HDSF system is located at Iron Mountain. Each of the microscopes is currently equipped with a Toshiba 3CCD camera, which, along with improved software, allows transmission of higher-resolution dynamic (real-time) or static (still) images compared with the camera and software described previously [4, 10, 14]. In addition to microscopes and associated computer units, all sites have gross examination stations and/or document readers to capture both dynamic and static macroscopic images of surgical pathology or autopsy specimens, microbiology culture plates, or other items. An interface has been developed that allows storage of static pathology images within the electronic medical record system of the VHA. Such images are available to clinicians using computer workstations. In 2001, software was upgraded to allow multiple sites within VISN 12 to connect simultaneously. Previously, the system had been configured for point-to-point communications only.

3.2
Primary Diagnosis and Clinical Consultation in Surgical Pathology

The robotic telepathology connection between the Iron Mountain and Milwaukee VAMCs has been used since mid-1996 to render over 9,000 diagnoses in routine surgical pathology. Dr. Choi has personally signed out almost 4,000 cases using telepathology. Typically, we perform up to ten frozen sections per year. Diagnostic accuracy (clinically significant) of approximately 99.7% has been achieved in nondeferred cases [12]. In our system, pathologists are given the option to defer diagnosis to routine light microscopy if the case is difficult or requires special stains not performed on-site at Iron Mountain or if the

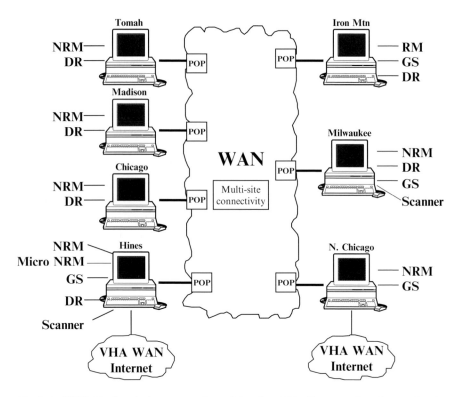

Fig. 3.2. VISN 12 telepathology network as of October 2007. Computer-based control units are present at all sites. A robotic microscope (RM) is located at Iron Mountain. All other sites have nonrobotic microscopes (NRM). Because of the large distance between the main laboratory and the microbiology laboratory at Hines, we have installed a separate nonrobotic telepathology unit in both locations, as shown. Individual sites have gross stations (GS), document readers (DR), and/or scanners, as needed. Each telepathology unit is connected to the wide area network (WAN) through a connection known as a "point of presence" (POP). Multiple sites can connect simultaneously (multisite connectivity). Through connections at Hines and North Chicago, all sites can connect to the Veterans Hospital Administration Intranet. This figure was modified with permission from one published previously [14]

additional time required to read slides by telepathology is felt to be too great a burden, based on the daily staffing [11, 12]. An important consideration of the robotic HDSF system we use is that for the inexperienced telepathologist, it can take three to five times longer to read a case by telepathology than by routine light microscopy [11, 25]. With experience, however, the time to make a diagnosis typically decreases [11, 25].

The ability of pathologists to see the gross tissue in large specimens, such as colectomy specimens, is critical to their ability to make accurate diagnoses. Since the inception of the Iron Mountain–Milwaukee telepathology service, we have used a tele-gross tissue examination system [2, 3], to allow pathologists to view live images of gross specimens in real time, if necessary. In addition, the system allows annotation of digitized gross images. Initially, pathologists used the system routinely to view gross images. However, as the experience of the on-site pathologists' assistant (DLR) increased, and resultant pathologist confidence increased, pathologists now typically only view the annotated digital images at the time of sign out. Telepathology has been described at other VHA facilities outside of VISN 12 as well [7, 27].

An important lesson we have learned is that for telepathology to be successful in the absence of an on-site pathologist, a well-trained individual knowledgeable in the significance, description, and processing of gross specimens must be present on-site. We recommend that such an individual be board certified as a pathologists' assistant. In this regard, Mr. Daniel Recla, a coauthor of this chapter, is a medical technologist, who in mid-1995 served as supervisor of the blood bank, hematology, and microbiology sections of the Iron Mountain VAMC laboratory, which at that time had 13 employees. After receiving on-the-job training provided by the on-site Iron Mountain pathologist prior to the pathologist's retirement and by pathologists in Milwaukee, Mr. Recla successfully passed the examination for board certification as a pathologists' assistant by the American Association of Pathologists' Assistants (AAPA). Currently, Mr. Recla serves as pathologists' assistant, laboratory information manager, and lead medical technologist at the Iron Mountain VAMC. Milwaukee pathologists have repeatedly expressed to the senior author that if they did not have confidence in the on-site pathologists' assistant, they would refuse to sign out cases using telepathology. Mr. Recla serves as eyes, ears, and even nose for the Milwaukee pathologists. His ability to communicate concisely with surgeons in Iron Mountain and pathologists in Milwaukee has been and continues to be one of the most important factors in the success of the Iron Mountain–Milwaukee telepathology initiative.

Table 3.1 emphasizes that, to this day, the most extensive use of telepathology in VISN 12 occurs between Iron Mountain and Milwaukee, located just over 220 miles apart. Of interest, while Milwaukee pathologists also provide surgical pathology, cytopathology, and autopsy pathology (North Chicago only) services to both Tomah and North Chicago, we have not implemented robotic telepathology systems at either of these sites. At Tomah, the decision to send fixed tissue directly to Milwaukee without implementing robotic telepathology was made based on the absence of inpatient surgery. Approximately 600 biopsies (primarily skin and gastrointestinal specimens) are obtained at Tomah annually. Cost savings were realized by closing the on-site histology laboratory at Tomah and sending cases to Milwaukee. Clinicians have expressed pleasure with the diagnostic services provided, and administrators have appreciated the cost savings. Nonrobotic telepathology (in which the individual at the remote site directs the images being shown) is available should the need arise to view

Table 3.1. Current uses of telepathology in VISN 12

Use	Remote site	Hub site
Anatomic pathology		
Frozen section diagnosis	IM	Milwaukee
Routine primary diagnosis	IM	Milwaukee
Clinical consultation	IM, Tomah, and NC	Milwaukee
Autopsy conferences	IM and NC	Milwaukee
Clinical conferences	IM, Tomah, and NC	Milwaukee
Consultation	All sites	Milwaukee and Hines
Digital imaging	All sites	None needed
Clinical pathology		
Microbiology, diagnostic	IM, Tomah, NC, Madison, and Chicago	Milwaukee and Hines
Microbiology, teaching	NC	Milwaukee
Peripheral blood smears	IM, Tomah, and NC	Milwaukee
Body fluids	IM, Tomah, and NC	Milwaukee
Clinical conferences	IM and NC	Milwaukee

Remote site refers to the site sending images to a consulting (hub) site. *IM* Iron Mountain, *NC* North Chicago

a gross specimen at Tomah from Milwaukee in real time. At North Chicago VAMC (located 56 mile from Milwaukee), we have maintained a small histology laboratory in which uncomplicated tissues are processed and slides generated. Between 1990 and 2006, inpatient surgery was not performed at North Chicago VAMC. However, in mid-2006, with the completion of the first phase of consolidation between North Chicago VAMC and Great Lakes Naval Hospital (located 3 mile apart), Navy surgeons began performing limited general inpatient surgery at the North Chicago VAMC. At the present time, Milwaukee VAMC pathologists, rather than Navy pathologists, are responsible for signing out such cases. The occasional large specimens generated (i.e., colectomies, hysterectomies, and others) are fixed at North Chicago and transported on one of two daily courier runs to Milwaukee. Frozen sections and CT-guided fine needle aspirations are occasionally performed at North Chicago VAMC. Rather than using telepathology, a pathologist from the Navy or Milwaukee VAMC travels to the North Chicago laboratory. Reasons for not implementing robotic telepathology on-site at North Chicago include absence of a qualified pathologists' assistant who can multitask as a medical technologist and relatively close proximity to Milwaukee with two courier runs daily.

Currently, pathologists from Milwaukee travel to Iron Mountain and North Chicago to perform autopsies. Digitized images of key gross findings are generated using handheld digital cameras or gross tissue workstations. Upon completion of the autopsy, digitized images can be sent electronically to the attending clinician. In addition, autopsy conferences are conducted at Iron Mountain by the pathologist (from a distance) who performed the autopsy using digital images.

3.3
Diagnosis and Consultation in Clinical Pathology

In clinical pathology, telepathology is used at virtually all sites in diagnostic microbiology to help diagnose rare or interesting infections and/or microorganisms. The successful application of telemicrobiology has resulted from the leadership of supervisors at Milwaukee and Hines, the two core microbiology laboratories for VISN 12, to which microbiology specimens from the five primary laboratories are transported. Clinical microbiology has been consolidated to Milwaukee core laboratory from the Tomah, Madison, and North Chicago laboratories. While bacteriology has remained on-site at Iron Mountain, workload in parasitology, mycology, and mycobacteriology has been consolidated from that site to Milwaukee. Similarly, microbiology workload from VA Chicago has been consolidated to the core laboratory at Hines. Gram stains are performed and read at the primary laboratories in VISN 12; then culture plates are set up and transported in temperature-controlled portable incubators to the core laboratories. Dynamic and static images of culture plates and smears can be shared between the primary laboratories and the core laboratories as needed, using the telepathology system. Of interest, core laboratories occasionally have the opportunity to view dynamic images of the motility or other features of viable clinical microorganisms in wet fresh preparations viewed microscopically in an attempt to assist in their identification. Weekly telemicrobiology conferences are conducted between North Chicago and Milwaukee, in part to help support the Infectious Diseases Fellowship Program at North Chicago. In addition, nonrobotic telepathology can be used at Iron Mountain and Tomah to show Gram stains, peripheral blood smears, and body fluids to pathologists at Milwaukee, to provide timely results to clinicians. Finally, multiple clinical conferences are provided by Milwaukee pathologists to clinicians at both Iron Mountain and North Chicago. At least one feasibility study of telemicrobiology has been published [22].

Telepathology is an essential networking tool in the consolidated VISN 12 Pathology and Laboratory Medicine Service Line in which clinical laboratories are separated by distances of up to 320 mile. In our experience, telepathology has proven useful not only in surgical pathology, the area in which we initially perceived its value, but also in all areas in the clinical laboratory in which viewing of macroscopic and/or microscopic images is important. In VISN 12, telepathology is used not only by pathologists but also by skilled technologists in areas such as microbiology and hematology, as both a diagnostic and an educational tool. As we have described previously, in the right environment, telepathology can be cost effective compared with maintaining an on-site pathologist at a remote site [1]. Others support this contention [21]. In VISN 12, the cost of the hardware and software comprising the telepathology network shown in Fig. 3.2 has been leveraged against a reduction in pathologist salaries. Between 1996 and 1999, we reduced the number of pathologist full-time equivalents from 32 to approximately 20, due, in large part, to the implementation of the telepathology network.

It must be noted, however, that implementation of telepathology has not completely eliminated the need for pathologists and technologists to travel between sites in VISN 12. For example, the VISN 12 chief pathologist and administrative directors of the northern and southern tiers of the service line travel weekly to other sites to attend medical executive committee meetings, administrative meetings, laboratory staff meetings, and clinical conferences and/or to perform autopsies. Although it is possible that several of these functions could be "attended" by videoconference or teleconference, we believe that it is essential to interact face to face with clinicians and key hospital administrators at multiple sites to promote mutual respect and understanding. In general, chiefs of staff, clinicians, and hospital administrators have complimented the high quality and improved cost effectiveness of the consolidated pathology services provided in VISN 12.

3.4
Future Developments in Telepathology

We hope to upgrade our telepathology image database to one that is searchable using key phrases. Our existing database is searchable only by patient name or other demographic data. However, at the present time, we cannot search for all cases showing a specific type of pathology. The upgrade is available commercially and we hope to have funding available for this improvement soon.

By the year 2010, we expect that the volume of surgical and clinical pathology specimens requiring review by a pathologist will increase sufficiently that the VHA and/or Department of the Navy will station at least one pathologist on-site at the North Chicago VAMC. When this change occurs, the telepathology system currently in place will allow the pathologist to consult with other pathologists in VISN 12.

Thinking more broadly, what we really need to achieve in telepathology is the same resolution of live images on the computer screen that we can obtain using the light microscope. Such is not the case at present. Much of surgical pathology involves scanning of slides at low magnification to determine whether pathology is present. Higher magnification can then be used to confirm the presence of pathology and to determine the nature of the pathologic process. While the imaging capabilities of the HDSF system we have employed for over 10 years are good and have improved over time, pathologists using the system universally agree that the resolution of live images obtained using low magnification by HDSF telepathology is not quite as good as that observed when looking directly through a light microscope at the same magnification. As a result, slide scanning by telepathology has to be performed at higher magnification, resulting in longer times required for slide viewing. Increased resolution could potentially be achieved by transmitting more digital information per unit time (resulting in increased telecommunications costs) or perhaps by some novel methods. Whole slide imaging is another method potentially allowing greater resolution at low magnification [16, 17]. For low-volume services such as that at Iron Mountain VAMC, the delay involved in digitizing routine slides would not appreciably reduce the turn around time for reports. However, the delay in digitizing slides for frozen sections would likely prove excessive. Methods are being developed to more rapidly digitize entire slides [26]. We need to compare image quality achievable using the current HDSF system with that available using whole slide imaging. An important question, of course, will be whether the perceived improved quality, and presumably reduced pathologist time spent screening slides, would warrant the investment in whole slide imaging technology.

In summary, telepathology serves as in integral service component within VISN 12 of the United States VHA. Telepathology has proven beneficial within other hospital systems as well [5, 6, 18–20, 28]. An important benefit of telepathology at rural sites is provision of access to the opinions of multiple medical school-affiliated anatomic and clinical pathologists in real time, since it can be difficult to recruit pathologists in rural settings due to geographic isolation and cost constraints. By increasing access to pathologists and technologists within the Pathology and Laboratory Medicine Service Line, telepathology networking has become an essential strategic component of the VISN 12 staffing and budget plan.

3.5
Summary

- Telepathology involves the sending and viewing of video and digitized images for the purpose of rendering primary or consultative diagnoses by pathologists at a distance.
- Robotic telepathology, in which a hub-site pathologist located at a distance from the remote-site microscope is able to control slide movement and adjust magnification, focus, and lighting, has been in place continuously between the Iron Mountain and Milwaukee VAMCs since 1996. Images are viewed on a computer screen.
- For telepathology to function effectively in the absence of an on-site pathologist, we recommend that a board-certified pathologists' assistant be available at the remote site.
- Nonrobotic HDSF telepathology systems are present at all six VISN 12 hospital laboratories other than Iron Mountain.
- Applications of telepathology include frozen sections and routine paraffin-embedded tissue, autopsy pathology, microbiology, peripheral blood smears, body fluids, and clinical conferences.
- Implementation of telepathology has allowed VISN 12 to provide a single standard of accurate and timely pathology and laboratory medicine service, even at small hospitals that lack an on-site pathologist.
- In the right environment, telepathology can be a cost-effective tool.
- The most important need in telepathology is to improve resolution of live (dynamic) images, especially at low magnification, to facilitate more rapid slide review, similar to that performed by standard light microscopy.

Acknowledgment

We thank Mr. Mark Maticek for providing the figures.

References

1. Agha Z, Weinstein RS, Dunn BE (1999) Cost minimization analysis of a dynamic robotic telepathology service implemented within the Department of Veterans Affairs. Am J Clin Pathol 112:470–478
2. Almagro UA, Dunn BE, Choi H, Recla DL, Weinstein RS (1996) The gross pathology workstation: an essential component of a dynamic-robotic telepathology system. Cell Vision 3:470–473

 3. Almagro UA, Dunn BE, Choi H, Chejfec G, Recla DL (1998) Telepathology in the VA Healthcare System: the VISN 12 experience. Fed Practitioner 15:55–65
 4. Almagro UA, Dunn BE, Choi H, Recla DL (1998) Telepathology. Am J Surg Pathol 22:1161–1163
 5. Brauchli K, Oberli H, Hurwitz N, et al (2004) Diagnostic telepathology: long-term experience of a single institution. Virch Arch 444:403–409
 6. Chorneyko K, Giesler R, Sabatino D, et al (2002) Telepathology for routine light microscopic and frozen section diagnosis. Am J Clin Pathol 117:783–790
 7. Dawson PJ, Johnson JG, Edgemon LJ, Brand CR, Hall E, Van Buskirk GF (2000) Outpatient frozen sections by telepathology in a Veterans Administration medical center. Hum Pathol 31:786–788
 8. Dunn BE, Chejfec G, Weinstein RS (1996) Progress toward development of a full service telepathology-based laboratory. Cell Vision 3:463–466
 9. Dunn BE, Choi H, Almagro UA (1996) Dynamic-robotic telepathology on-line: summary of first 200 cases. Cell Vision 3:467–469
10. Dunn BE, Almagro UA, Choi H, Recla DL, Weinstein RS (1997) Use of telepathology for routine surgical pathology in a test bed in the Department of Veterans Affairs. Telemed J 3:1–10
11. Dunn BE, Almagro UA, Choi H, et al (1997) Dynamic-robotic telepathology: Department of Veterans Affairs feasibility study. Hum Pathol 28:8–12
12. Dunn BE, Choi H, Almagro UA, Recla DL, Weinstein RS (1999) Routine surgical telepathology in the Department of Veterans Affairs: experience-related improvements in pathologist performance in 2200 cases. Telemed J 5:323–337
13. Dunn BE, Choi H, Almagro UA, Recla DL, Davis CW (2000) Telepathology networking in VISN 12 of the Veterans Health Administration. Telemed J e-Health 3:349–354
14. Dunn BE, Choi H, Almagro UA, Recla DL (2001) Combined robotic and nonrobotic telepathology as an integral service component of a geographically dispersed laboratory network. Hum Pathol 32:1300–1303
15. Eide TJ, Nordrum I (1994) Current status of telepathology. APMIS 102:881–890
16. Glatz-Krieger K, Glatz D, Mihatsch MJ (2003) Virtual slides: high-quality demand, physical limitations, and affordability. Hum Pathol 34:968–974
17. Ho J, Parwani AV, Jukic DM, Yagi Y, Anthony L, Gilbertson JR (2006) Use of whole slide imaging in surgical pathology quality assurance: design and pilot validation studies. Hum Pathol 7:322–331
18. Hutarew G, Dandachi N, Strasser F, Prokop E, Dietze O (2003) Two-year evaluation of telepathology. J Telemed Telecare 9:194–199
19. Kaplan KJ, Burgess JR, Sandberg GD, Myers CP, Bigott TR, Greenspan RB (2002) Use of robotic telepathology for frozen-section diagnosis: a retrospective trial of a telepathology system for intraoperative consultation. Modern Pathol 15:1197–1204
20. Kayser K, Kayser G, Radziszowski D, Oehmann A (2004) New developments in digital pathology: from telepathology to virtual pathology laboratory. Stud Health Technol Inform 105:61–69
21. Leong AS, Leong FJ (2005) Strategies for laboratory cost containment and for pathologist shortage: centralised pathology laboratories with microwave-stimulated histoprocessing and telepathology. Pathology 37:5–9
22. McLaughlin WJ, Schifman RB, Ryan KJ, et al (1998) Telemicrobiology: feasibility study. Telemed J 3:11–17
23. Weinstein RS, Bloom KJ, Rozek LS (1987) Telepathology and the networking of pathology diagnostic services. Arch Pathol Lab Med 111:646–652

24. Weinstein RS, Dunn BE, Graham AR (1997) Telepathology networks as models for studying telemedicine services. New Med 1:235–241
25. Weinstein RS, Descour MR, Laing C, et al (2001) Telepathology overview: from concept to implementation. Hum Pathol 32:1283–1299
26. Weinstein RS, Descour MR, Liang C, et al (2004) An array microscope for ultrarapid virtual slide processing and telepathology. Design, fabrication, and validation study. Hum Pathol 35:1303–1314
27. Weisz-Carrington P, Blount M, Kipreos B, et al (1999) Telepathology between Richmond and Beckley Veterans Affairs Hospitals: report on the first 1000 cases. Telemed J 5:367–373
28. Williams BH, Mullick FG, Butler DR, Herring RF, O'leary TJ (2001) Clinical evaluation of an international static image-based telepathology service. Hum Pathol 32:1309–1317

4

Teleneuropathology

Georg Hutarew

Neuropathology, the branch of medicine concerned with diseases of the central and peripheral nervous system, diagnoses open or stereotactic primary or secondary biopsies of surgical specimens to determine the presence, course, or extent of a disease. The specimens must be transported from the neurosurgical operating room to a Department of Neuropathology. If there is a large distance between the operating room in the Neurosurgical Department and the Department of Neuropathology, the following possibilities exist:

- Neuropathologists visit the peripheral department once or twice a week and observe intraoperative diagnosing.
- A telepathology system can connect both departments via the Internet [13, 26].
- A combination of both, with doctors in training or surgeons doing the specimen workup under the video guidance of an experienced neuropathologist.

The following technical systems are used for teleneuropathology:

1. Microscope with digital camera
2. Microscope with video camera, with or without robotic functions
3. Automated slide scanners
4. Systems similar to microscopes

Software programs permit remote control of all system functions from a distance.

4.1
Available Systems

4.1.1
Light Microscopes

Light microscopes with digital cameras make digital images of histological slides. The cameras are mounted on the microscope with an ocular tube or a C-mount. The images can be sent as email attachments [6, 14, 22, 31].

4.1.2
Scanner Systems

Scanner systems (Aperio Scanscope, USA, Hamamatsu, Japan, Zeiss, Germany) scan histological slides at preset magnifications (200× or 400×) and produce virtual slides. These are stored on servers and can be viewed with special viewer software. A software program performs all functions of a light microscope. Virtual microscopy can be done on screens at any distance [14, 17].

4.1.3
Robotic Microscopes

Light microscopes equipped with a motorized stage and a video camera can be used with remote software at any distance and with all functions. The observer can perform conventional light microscopy or virtual microscopy at any distance. Stitching software enables these systems to produce virtual slides [1, 13, 17, 26, 31].

4.1.4
Systems Similar to Microscopes

These inexpensive systems are similar to conventional microscopes with scanning stages (Leica DMD108, Germany) or are a fusion of a PC and a microscope (Nikon Coolscope, Japan). Both provide remote microscopy as a small robotic microscope. These depend on the use of screens as these have no oculars.

Teleneuropathology systems can be used for:

1. Intraoperative frozen section diagnosis
2. Second-opinion diagnosis
3. Collections of rare entities or teaching cases
4. Multicenter studies
5. Specialist discussion [29]

4.2
Intraoperative Frozen Section Diagnosis

4.2.1
General

Intraoperative diagnosis in neuropathology serves two purposes. On the one hand, primary diagnoses have to determine the nature of a lesion, namely inflammatory or reactive vs. benign or malignant. Additionally, the patholo-gist must decide if it is necessary to take material for further microbiological, electron microscopic, or other special examination. On the other hand, the neuropathologist identifies the nature of resection margins, whether the lesion was excised completely or not, although en bloc resections are rare in neuro-surgical specimens.

These diagnoses have great influence on the subsequent surgical or conserv-ative therapeutic procedures. Therefore, only technical components of high-quality and professional standards that ensure stability and high reliability can be used [10].

A teleneuropathology link makes sense only if the distance between the neurosurgical operating room, the neuropathological laboratory, and the neu-ropathologist is so far that delivering specimens by messenger or ambulance would take too long [26]. We evaluated mean time for diagnosis of frozen sec-tions with conventional light microscopy (11 min) and with telemicroscopy (26 min). A telepathology system should be considered if transporting speci-mens takes more than 15 min [13].

4.2.2
Equipment for Frozen Section Diagnosis

4.2.2.1
Gross Examination

We use a one-chip camera (KPDA20AP Hitachi, Japan) with a resolution of 765 × 580 pixels, mounted on a repro station with a high-quality objective (Fig. 4.1).

Software adapts the transmitted video stream to the bandwidth by changing the compression rate or resolution. We diagnose gross examination even at a reso-lution of 320 × 160 pixels. The neuropathologist can navigate the remote camera (zoom function, illumination, and focusing) from a distance via the Internet (Fig. 4.2). If the bandwidth is small, software has to provide more subtle functions. Webcams of the newest generation with resolutions of 640 × 480 pixels video stream and the ability to provide snapshots or stereoscopic systems can be used for recognizing distinct and delicate surface structures of specimens [12].

4.2.2.2
Microscope

We use a robotic microscope Eclipse 1000E (Nikon, Japan) with magni-fications ranging from 5× to 630×, a motorized scanning stage (Märzhäuser, Germany), and a three-chip video camera, HV-C20A (Hitachi, Japan) with a

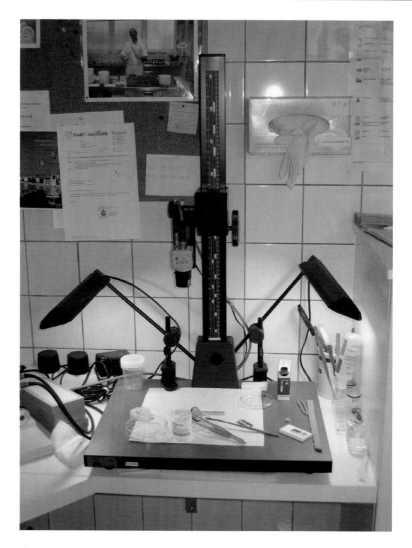

Fig. 4.1. Gross examination in neuropathology laboratory

resolution of 765 × 560 pixels (Fig. 4.3). For a long time, this camera was the state of the art for such systems. All microscope functions (changing magnification, focusing, illumination, and scanning stage movements) can be remotely controlled by the diagnosing neuropathologist from a distance via the Internet [15].

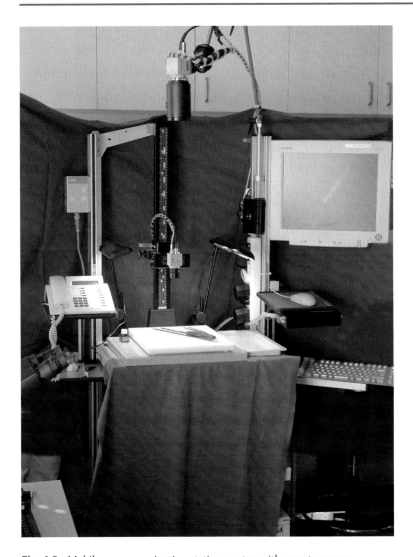

Fig. 4.2. Mobile gross examination station, on top with remote camera

4.2.2.3
Telepathology Software

A software program provides all functions for gross and microscopic remote examination in teleneuropathology. The program is stored on a PC with server functions. Pathologists can log onto the server, view or review stored sessions, and maneuver the microscope. The program regulates three different video streams and permits discussion with the help of pointers and text annotations

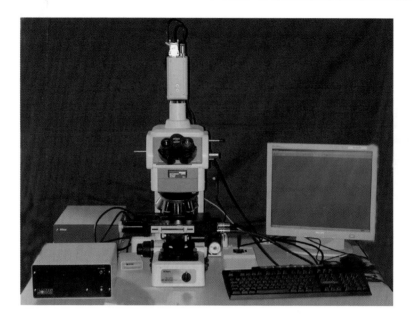

Fig. 4.3. Robotic microscope E1000 Nikon, motorized Märzhäuser scanning stage, and electronic boxes

during an established connection. Moreover, the program has a videoconferencing module (Fig. 4.4).

4.2.2.4
Diagnosis

The workplace where the neuropathologist makes his/her diagnosis is equipped with a PC with sufficient performance for the software, has an excellent graphics card, and screens with excellent image and color quality. The telepathology viewer controls macroscopy and microscopy. If allowed by the security system, the neuropathologist can log onto the hospital information system to consult the electronic patient data (Fig. 4.5).

4.2.2.5
Laboratory Equipment

Laboratory equipment for teleneuropathology is often underestimated with regard to cost. A laboratory technician is needed to cut and stain material during frozen section diagnosis. Quality of slides influences diagnostic quality, because telemicroscopy systems have problems with artifacts when screening thick or strongly stained slides. To stay in practices, a laboratory technician must maintain a minimal frequency with intraoperative cases.

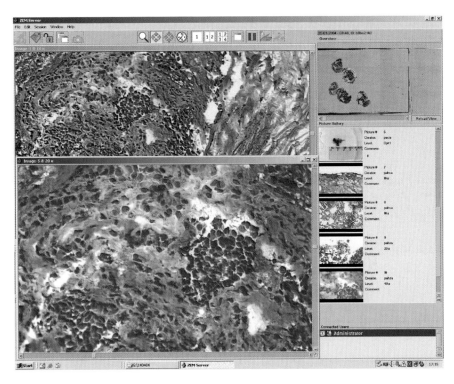

Fig. 4.4. Screenshot with two image fields on the left, overview; picture gallery of macroscopic and microscopic examination and connected users on the right

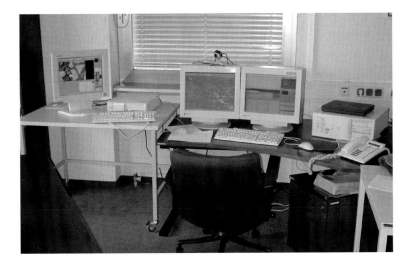

Fig. 4.5. Diagnosing station of the neuropathologist

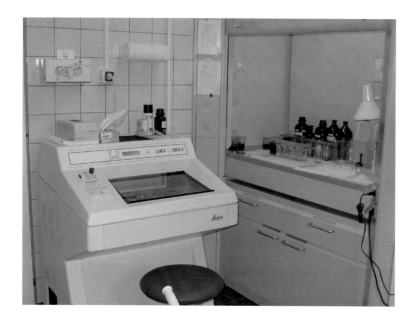

Fig. 4.6. Leica cryostat microtome

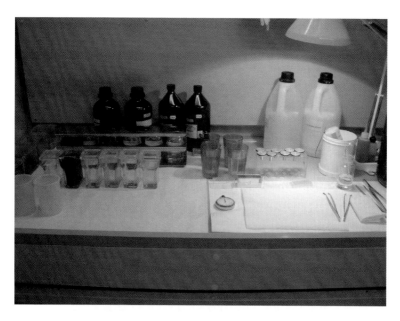

Fig. 4.7. Material for staining frozen section slides

An expensive cryostat microtome (Fig. 4.6) must be available, as well as a place for staining (Fig. 4.7). Some neurosurgical departments restrict operations with frozen section diagnosis to 1 or 2 days a week.

The robotic microscope, the macroscopic station, and the PC server must be serviced and monitored by technicians who can solve their problems and restore the system when necessary.

4.2.3
Sequence of Frozen Sections

The neuropathologist must know the patient's identity, age, sex, anamnesis, pretreatment, lesion localization, neuroradiological findings, and the planned surgical procedure before diagnosing specimens. These data can be sent by fax or email, or the neuropathologist can access the hospital information system to consult the patient's medical file.

When performing a craniotomy, the neurosurgeon in the operating room should be connected with the neuropathologist by means of video and telephone link. The neuropathologist can view the surgical field in situ and discuss the gathering of specimens with the surgeon.

Neuropathological specimens are small and delicate. For open and stereotactic biopsies, specimens must be taken and the subsequent careful workup must be performed according to the highest standards, to ensure excellent diagnostic quality.

The specimens taken during surgery are brought to the neuropathology laboratory, which should be located as near as possible to the operating room. Each specimen is given an ID number for further identification. The material is placed on the macroscopic station, and the neuropathologist views the specimen by video link. The neuropathologist uses annotations, i.e., pointers and circles, to show the laboratory technician which part of the specimen the neuropathologist wants for smear preparation and which portion for frozen section.

The smear preparation is stained (methyl blue) and placed under the robotic microscope (Fig. 4.8). An overview image is done at 0.5× magnification and the diagnostic areas are identified. These are scanned with light microscopy, and ideally the diagnosis is established.

Meanwhile, the laboratory technician has frozen, cut, and stained the histological slides with hematoxylin eosin. The slide is placed under the microscope, an overview image is made, and the slide is viewed as usual (Fig. 4.9). The diagnosis is established and given to the surgeon. This should be done by telephone link to allow discussion between the neuropathologist and the surgeon. This prevents misunderstandings and permits medical discrepancies to be correlated.

Our speech connections are via telephone, with the laboratory technician using a headset and wireless connection and the diagnosing neuropathologist a hands-free telephone. Telephone connections are independent of the computer connections and function regardless of network or computer problems.

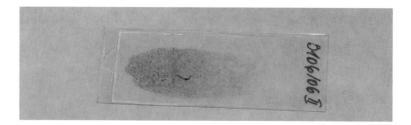

Fig. 4.8. The smear preparation is stained (methyl blue) and placed under the robotic microscope

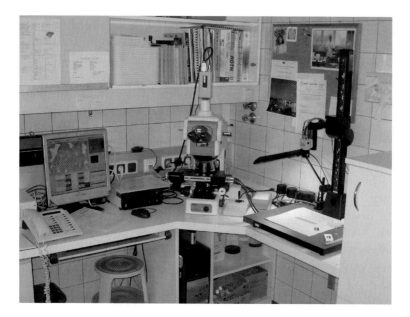

Fig. 4.9. Actual setup of the neuropathology laboratory. The smear preparation is stained (methyl blue) and placed under the robotic microscope (Fig. 4.8). An overview image is done at 0.5× magnification and the diagnostic areas are identified. These are scanned with light microscopy, and ideally the diagnosis is established

Not merely for reasons of quality assessment, the entire surgical specimen should be sent to the laboratory that previously diagnosed the frozen section. The specimens are routinely worked up and diagnosed as usual. Comparison of the slides with telemicroscopy and light microscopy is a good training for viewers and a good teaching aid.

The system records all data from the telemicroscopy sessions and stores them on a server, i.e., .avi for the video stream and .jpeg for macroscopic and histological examination. Documentation of the sessions and all areas viewed during intraoperative diagnosis can be helpful for forensic reasons.

4.2.4
Statistical Evaluation 2000–2007

We introduced our telepathology system between 2000 and 2002 and conducted a study parallel thereto [11]. In that study, we diagnosed 342 intraoperative frozen sections with specimens typical for surgical pathology in our department. Doctors and laboratory technicians learned the method and familiarized themselves with telemicroscopy. Experiences were integrated into the workflow and telemicroscopy software. Intraoperative diagnoses and teleneuropathological diagnoses – both of which entail brief macroscopic examination but extensive cytological and histological examination – took between 16 and 25 min (mean value). At the end of the study, we had halved the time required for diagnosis.

Between 2002 and 2005, we diagnosed for a neurosurgical department 2 km away from us; we conducted 343 teleneuropathological intraoperative diagnoses [13]. From 2005 to 2007, the Department of Neuropathology at Vienna Medical University carried out 265 frozen section diagnoses using the same telepathology system and the same laboratory equipment and staff as in Salzburg.

Our connection in Salzburg had a bandwidth of 38 Mb s^{-1}; the connection to the neuropathology department in Vienna started at 1 Mb s^{-1} and ultimately had 5 Mb s^{-1}. Our telepathology system has the capacity to handle 1 Mb s^{-1}. One of the reasons why the system was a little slower when connected to Vienna was because of the security architecture.

The mean time needed for frozen section diagnosis was 26 min (range 15–40 min), macroscopic examination 3 min, staining 4.2 min, smear diagnosis 5.4 min, and histological diagnosis 10.7 min [10, 13, 24].

The neuropathologists in Vienna originally started with telemicroscopic diagnosing. The mean time needed for frozen section diagnosis was 32.6 min, measured from arrival of the specimens in the laboratory until the diagnosis was given to the neurosurgeon. The first 100 diagnoses took 38.68 min (mean value), whereas the following 100 diagnoses took 30.12 min (mean value), and the last group took 26.22 min. Interestingly, time required for diagnosis in all groups (surgical pathology and teleneuropathology) leveled at 26 min under optimal circumstances, so to speak at system speed.

Time needed for cytological and histological examination was 23.46 min in the first group, 16.93 min in the second, and 15.9 min in the third group.

Interestingly, time needed for cutting and staining was also reduced, namely to 15.22, 13.12, and 10.32 min [13]. Workflow was optimized, with routine and teamwork proving to be immensely advantageous, especially in telemedicine (Table 4.1) [10, 28].

The diagnostic criteria in teleneuropathology and surgical pathology differ. For a craniotomy, it is necessary to know whether diagnostic material was sent and whether the lesion was hit. Some lesions can be diagnosed immediately as meningiomas, whereas glial tumors require careful grading during surgery, with the exception that an unmistakable glioblastoma can be identified.

We compared light microscopy and telemicroscopy by giving slides from frozen section diagnoses to the same neuropathologist months later for him/ her to review with light microscopy. Time needed for diagnosis was compared. Smear preparations took 11 times longer and histological slides 16 times longer with our telemicroscopy system than with light microscopy, whereby it should not be forgotten that our telemicroscopy system meanwhile is 7 years old. Our system needed 35 s to produce the overview image of a slide, a time in which a diagnostician working under ideal circumstances can establish a diagnosis with light microscopy [7, 13, 17, 24].

During the first teleneuropathology study, we experienced minor technical problems in 6% of cases, which delayed the time required for diagnosis by not more than 4 min. System reliability was 100%, meaning that we were able to render a diagnosis in every case.

The telepathology link from Salzburg to Vienna posed many minor technical problems in 9% of cases, similar to those shown in Table 4.2. In addition, we also experienced misunderstandings because of communication problems.

Table 4.1. Mean values with telepathology [13]

Frozen sections	Mean time (min)	Macroscopy (min)	Staining (min)	Smear (min)	Histology (min)
0–342	26	3	4.2	5.4	10.7
343–443	38.68	6.3	8.8	7.8	15.59
444–544	30.12	5.46	7.65	5.6	11.25
545–610	26.22	4.3	6.01	5.3	10.56

Mean accuracy of diagnosis was 97.6% [13]. An international comparison reported 92–100% accuracy [5, 17, 18, 28]

Table 4.2. Technical problems experienced during 4 years of telepathology [13]

Description of error 2002–2005	Occurrence
Minor software problems, i.e., loss of some navigation functions	Often
Deviation between virtual position and real position on slide	Often
Freezing of video streams	Often
Network problems	Sometimes
Missing overview image	Twice
Joystick of scanning stage did not respond	Sometimes
Microscope malfunction (electric macroslider)	Once
Malfunction in electronic box of scanning stage	Once

Neuropathologists complained that the system worked too slowly with slow video streams and snapshots taking too long; these were most often interpreted as network problems. After checking the system, we found that the local storage capacity was overrun and solved the problem by deleting old files from the active memory. In another case, diagnosis was impossible because the system could not establish a connection. This was interpreted as a software failure. A system check showed that the IP addresses had been changed without us being informed.

A logical and organized structure must be created when diagnosing from a distance [20]. This is especially important when several telemedical connections are operated with different departments. A chat connection with Webcams might be helpful in some cases.

4.3
Second-Opinion Diagnosis and Specialist Discussion

If a diagnosis cannot be established or the clinicians do not accept the diagnosis in the case of therapy-refractory patients, another diagnosis must be obtained from a specialized center. Slides and paraffin-embedded material are sent by post, and the reference center examines the case and suggests a diagnosis [27]. This procedure can take up to 2 weeks.

Telemicroscopy systems can reduce time for reference diagnosis, but they are not widely accepted. We lack standardization and an accepted organization for reference diagnosing.

4.3.1
Digital Camera

It is easy to equip a microscope with a digital camera and send images as email attachments. It must be assured that the diagnostic areas are on the images. We find this to be an uncomplicated method that gives astonishingly good results [2, 16, 21–23].

4.3.2
Video Camera

A microscope equipped with a video camera, with or without remote control, is an excellent system. A pathologist who asks for a reference diagnosis is linked via Internet with a reference diagnostician who views the slide. In other words, this is a virtual digital discussion system.

It is a little more sophisticated if the reference diagnostician can remotely control the microscope and the scanning stage via the network. The diagnostician views the slide as if it was under his/her light microscope and decides whether he/she can do the diagnosis immediately or not. Snapshots and parts of the slides can be recorded for later review [15].

4.3.3
Robotic Microscope

Virtual slides produced with a robotic microscope or with a slide scanner can be stored on a server and presented to a diagnostician anywhere. The viewer examines the virtual case with special viewing software, whenever and how often the viewer wants. This system is perfect for pathologists, most of whom are quite impatient [1, 4].

The sending of slides and specimens can be reduced to those cases that require additional examination at specialized departments. The main disadvantage is the immense storage capacity needed, up to 3 GB per virtual slide, with many cases having up to 25 and more slides including immunohistochemical slides, 75 GB per case. The technical architecture of such a system is expensive and should rather be implemented at central hospitals or university departments than in peripheral departments.

4.4
Database with Virtual Slides

Many institutions and medical societies set up databases with collections of macroscopic and histological slides. Reference diagnoses, teaching cases for students or postgraduates, training for virtual microscopy and rapid call-up of stored cases within seconds and from anywhere are the advantages of this method. In intercenter studies, various viewers give their opinion on cases that are discussed. Results are analyzed and statistically evaluated. Slides of rare entities can be presented to several observers without damaging or using up rare material [3, 4, 9, 14, 32].

4.5
Data Protection

Hospital information systems and sensitive patient data have strict security clearance. The rooms for macroscopic examination and the microscope are locked, with access being accorded to authorized persons only. The hospital information system requires password-protected access, as does the telepathology software, which can connect only with computers that are entered to a connection file. We do not enter any patient data except an ID number, similar to the histological case number in traditional pathology. We turn on the system only when a session is running and a telephone connection is established. We do not use the 128-bit encryption module, because it slows down the whole system. All connected users are shown in a separate window, and other connections are blocked at that time.

Patient data were exchanged by fax or email. The files were split into various tiles during transfer and pieced together with special software. The neuropathologist gives the diagnosis to the neurosurgeon by telephone link. The Salzburg–Vienna connection crossed two hospital firewalls with VPN tunneling with a dedicated network line.

4.6
Discussion of Teleneuropathology

The main disadvantage of teleneuropathology is the long time needed for diagnosis as compared with light microscopy. Smear preparations for neuropathology pose special problems when using systems like ours. How long a diagnosis takes depends, in part, on the various pathologists, on their experience in telemicroscopy and light microscopy, and also on their personal work style. We evaluated (unpublished data) a factor of 3, meaning that the slowest diagnostician was three times slower than the fastest.

Times for cutting and staining differ from technician to technician, and a laboratory team that does not work well together further prolongs time to diagnosis. Accuracy of diagnosis does not correlate with time to diagnosis but depends on the diagnostician's experience. Cases with good diagnostic material take only a short time, whereas difficult cases, rare entities, or specimens consisting of poorly preserved material prolong time to diagnosis.

Neurosurgeons' workup of each case and their adherence to the highest standards when gathering surgical specimens are important for the diagnostic result. A direct in situ video connection between the operating room and the neuropathologist should be available for open biopsies. Quality depends on human factors such as experience, interest in the technique, struggle for successful diagnosis, and the conviction that telemedical diagnosing makes sense.

A department must choose software and hardware that agrees with its methodology. Requirements differ depending on local laws and the regulations for forensic documentation, e.g., the amount of patient data or annotations that must be recorded. The software should enable adaptation to the bandwidth, an important feature when diagnosing at long distance without a dedicated line. A computer and network administrator must be available for troubleshooting in case telepathology poses problems. If a telepathologist recognized problems correctly, time needed for diagnosis was not prolonged for more than 4 min during our study.

Security standards at modern hospitals restrict network strategies. On the one hand, telemedicine demands cooperation between pathologists and other departments, and on the other hand, hospitals restrict access to patient files to a small circle of authorized persons. Security systems slow telemedicine systems and, in the worst case, make them instable. Sometimes, it is easier to position the telemicroscopy server outside the firewall and to use the system only when a frozen section diagnosis has to be performed.

We anonymize each case by leaving patient data outside the system. We use a single ID number like the histological number on the slides in light microscopy. Transferring downsized neuroradiological or CT images is very important for the neuropathologist [25]. The neuropathologist does not make the radiological diagnosis, but he/she should be informed about lesion localization and size.

Telemedicine systems should give correct error messages to inform the user of problems and enable him/her to recognize errors and solve them. Unfortunately, we have not yet encountered such a program.

Copyright has become a problem for database systems. No one minds if images are used by third parties for studies or for teaching with no ulterior motive. Unfortunately, the scientific community loses sight of a selfless sharing of images, and business interests increasingly overshadow this idealistic concept.

Second-opinion diagnosing with telemedicine systems is also a legal issue, mainly in cases involving wrong diagnosis and especially when a patient suffers harm from wrong reference diagnosis. In general, second-opinion diagnoses from a reference center are deemed advice from a reference diagnostician to the requesting pathologist and can be quoted as such.

4.7
Future Aspects

It is our experience that telemedicine systems do not require an expensive microscope, a precision scanning stage, or a precision scanner. These cost too much [18]. Our software was programmed for small bandwidths but cannot utilize fast network connections.

Screening of large areas in cytological specimens like smear preparations in teleneuropathology takes too long and cannot be accelerated. Neither surgeons nor pathologists tolerate long times to diagnosis. Thus, time to diagnosis must be decreased until it approximates that of light microscopy.

A telemicroscopy system should do the following:

- Reduce transferred data volume.
- Utilize fastest Internet connections.
- Provide light and slim programming with modular technique, i.e., by using only what is really needed.
- Ensure continuity of software and hardware, i.e., new developments must integrate older systems with downward and upward compatibility.
- Be standardized so that different systems can communicate with each other.
- Provide uniformity of used symbols and short keys.
- Work with intuitive programming so that a user who is familiar with telemicroscopy can immediately use the system without first consulting a user manual.
- Have security standards that do not slow down systems.
- Have as few patient or insurance data as possible.
- Be integrated with department workflow.

We feel that such systems can be realized with a small microscope, a small but fast scanning stage, and a video camera. Video streams are compressed and transmitted in real time and allow slides to be screened. First tests have shown that such systems can be realized without undue effort [19]. As available bandwidth increases and costs decrease, we feel that our requirements are justified.

Screen development for histology should follow the strategy of increasing pixel number and decreasing screen size. Images are more brilliant and sharp. Our field of vision on the screen and under the microscope should be as similar as possible. Small displays might replace microscope oculars.

Although we have diagnosed on screens for years, we favor light microscopes and use them whenever possible. These are fast, are easy to handle, and provide a brilliance and highest quality better than any virtual microscopy system.

4.8
Summary

- Neuropathology, the branch of medicine concerned with diseases of the nervous system, diagnoses biopsies of surgical specimens to determine the presence, course, or extent of a disease.
- If there is a large distance between the operating room in the Neurosurgical Department and the Department of Neuropathology, a telepathology system can connect both departments via the Internet.
- Different technical systems are used for teleneuropathology, such as micro-scope with digital camera; microscope with video camera, with or without robotic functions; automated slide scanners; and innovative systems similar to microscopes.
- Teleneuropathology systems can be used for intraoperative frozen section diagnosis, second-opinion diagnosis, collections of rare entities or teaching cases, multicenter studies, and specialist discussion.
- Teleneuropathology is discussed in detail and future aspects of telemicros-copy are concluded, based on what we experienced with teleneuropathology during 7 years.

Appendix: Situation in Austria

Austria has a dense network of hospitals and pathology departments. Since there is, thus, no real need for telemicroscopy or teleneuropathology, these are not yet widely accepted. On the one hand, requesting help with a diagnosis via telemedicine is regarded as a sign of weakness by some pathologists. On the other hand, medical personnel are expected to work efficiently and meet chal-lenges. Pathology departments have to manage their own budget. As long as telemedicine and teleneuropathology take a long time and are not profitable, they will not find wide acceptance. Most telepathology links were set up to try out the new technology and rarely because they were needed.

Moreover, the legal situation is not clearly defined, but there is wide acceptance that telemicroscopy produces an expertise. Teleneuropathologists are experts who give advice to a requesting department [30].

To our knowledge, some telepathology connections are in operation for surgical pathology, but aside from ours there are no teleneuropathology systems in routine use. Efforts are occasionally made to establish telepathology connections with hospitals in the third world, mainly in cooperation with colleagues who studied in Austria or when an Austrian company builds or plans hospitals in other countries. Despite all discussion and the numerous technical and system deficits, we shall continue working with telemicroscopy and teleneuropathology [8].

Acknowledgments

Special thanks to C. Idriceanu, Salzburg University Clinics, Department of Neuropathology; H.U. Schlicker, MD, Salzburg University Clinics, Department of Pathology; F. Strasser, MD, Salzburg University Clinics, Department of Pathology; Professor J. Hainfellner, MD, Clinical Department of Neurology, Vienna Medical University; and Professor O. Dietze, MD, Salzburg University Clinics, Department of Pathology.

References

1. Costello SS, Johnston DJ, Dervan PA, O'Shea DG (2003) Development and evaluation of the virtual pathology slide: a new tool in telepathology. J Med Internet Res 5(2):e11
2. Crimmins D, Crooks D, Pickles A, Morris K (2005) Use of telepathology to provide rapid diagnosis of neurosurgical specimens. Neurochirurgie 51(2):84–88
3. Danda J, Juszkiewicz K, Leszczuk M, et al (2003) Medical video server construction. Pol J Pathol 54(3):197–204
4. Della Mea V (2005) Prerecorded telemedicine. J Telemed Telecare 11(6):276–284
5. Della Mea V, Demichelis F (2004) Accuracy of telepathology. J Telemed Telecare 10(2):123–124; author reply 124
6. Dennis T, Start RD, Cross SS (2005) The use of digital imaging, video conferencing, and telepathology in histopathology: a national survey. J Clin Pathol 58(3):254–258
7. Furness P (2007) A randomized controlled trial of the diagnostic accuracy of internet-based telepathology compared with conventional microscopy. Histopathology 50(2):266–273
8. Hartvigsen G, Johansen MA, Hasvold P, et al (2007) Challenges in telemedicine and eHealth: lessons learned from 20 years with telemedicine in Tromso. Stud Health Technol Inform 129:82–86
9. Helin H, Lundin M, Lundin J, et al (2005) Web-based virtual microscopy in teaching and standardizing Gleason grading. Hum Pathol 36(4):381–386

10. Horbinski C, Fine JL, Medina-Flores R, Yagi Y, Wiley CA (2007) Telepathology for intraoperative neuropathologic consultations at an academic medical center: a 5-year report. J Neuropathol Exp Neurol 66(8):750–759
11. Hutarew G, Dandachi N, Strasser F, Prokop E, Dietze O (2003) Two-year evaluation of telepathology. J Telemed Telecare 9(4):194–199
12. Hutarew G, Moser K, Dietze O (2004) Comparison of an auto-stereoscopic display and polarized stereoscopic projection for macroscopic pathology. J Telemed Telecare 10(4):206–213
13. Hutarew G, Schlicker HU, Idriceanu C, Strasser F, Dietze O (2006) Four years experience with teleneuropathology. J Telemed Telecare 12(8):387–391
14. Isabelle M, Teodorovic I, Oosterhuis JW, et al (2006) Virtual microscopy in virtual tumor banking. Adv Exp Med Biol 587:75–86
15. Kaplan KJ, Burgess JR, Sandberg GD, Myers CP, Bigott TR, Greenspan RB (2002) Use of robotic telepathology for frozen-section diagnosis: a retrospective trial of a telepathology system for intraoperative consultation. Mod Pathol 15(11):1197–1204
16. Lee ES, Kim IS, Choi JS, et al (2002) Practical telepathology using a digital camera and the Internet. Telemed J E Health 8(2):159–165
17. Li X, Liu J, Xu H, Gong E, et al (2007) A feasibility study of virtual slides in surgical pathology in China. Hum Pathol 38(12):1842–1848
18. Liang WY, Hsu CY, Lai CR, Ho DM, Chiang IJ (2008) Low-cost telepathology system for intraoperative frozen-section consultation: our experience and review of the literature. Hum Pathol 39(1):56–62
19. McKenna JK, Florell SR (2007) Cost-effective dynamic telepathology in the Mohs surgery laboratory utilizing iChat AV videoconferencing software. Dermatol Surg 33(1):62–68; discussion 68
20. Mireskandari M, Kayser G, Hufnagl P, Schrader T, Kayser K (2004) Teleconsultation in diagnostic pathology: experience from Iran and Germany with the use of two European telepathology servers. J Telemed Telecare 10(2):99–103
21. Nordrum I, Johansen M, Amin A, Isaksen V, Ludvigsen JA (2004) Diagnostic accuracy of second-opinion diagnoses based on still images. Hum Pathol 35(1):129–135
22. Papierz W, Szymas J, Danilewicz M, Della Mea V (2000) Determining the feasibility of diagnosing meningiomas using static teleneuropathy images transmitted electronically. Folia Neuropathol 38(1):39–42
23. Piccolo D, Soyer HP, Burgdorf W, et al (2002) Concordance between telepathologic diagnosis and conventional histopathologic diagnosis: a multiobserver store-and-forward study on 20 skin specimens. Arch Dermatol 138(1):53–58
24. Prayaga AK, Loya AC, Rao IS (2006) Telecytology – are we ready? J Telemed Telecare 12(6):319–320
25. Seidenari S, Pellacani G, Righi E, Di Nardo A (2004) Is JPEG compression of videomicroscopic images compatible with telediagnosis? Comparison between diagnostic performance and pattern recognition on uncompressed TIFF images and JPEG compressed ones. Telemed J E Health 10(3):294–303
26. Szymas J (2000) Technological requirements of teleneuropathological systems. Folia Neuropathol 38(2):85–88
27. Szymas J, Papierz W, Danilewicz M (2000) Real-time teleneuropathology for a second opinion of neurooncological cases. Folia Neuropathol 38(1):43–46
28. Szymas J, Wolf G, Papierz W, Jarosz B, Weinstein RS (2001) Online Internet-based robotic telepathology in the diagnosis of neuro-oncology cases: a teleneuropathology feasibility study. Hum Pathol 32(12):1304–1308

29. Walter GF (1999) Teleneuropathology: a means to improve the correctness of neuropathological diagnoses in clinical practice. Crit Rev Neurosurg 9(1):1–11
30. Walter GF, Walter KF (2003) Legal pitfalls in teleneuropathology. Methods Inf Med
42(3):255–259
31. Walter GF, Matthies HK, Brandis A, von Jan U (2000) Telemedicine of the future: teleneuropathology. Technol Health Care 8(1):25–34
32. Weinstein RS (2005) Innovations in medical imaging and virtual microscopy. Hum Pathol
36(4):317–319

Applications of Virtual Microscopy

P.H.J. Riegman, W.N.M. Dinjens, M.H.A. Oomen, W.F. Clotscher,
R.J.J.R. Scholte, W. Sjoerdsma, A.R.A. Riegman, and J.W. Oosterhuis

5.1
Introduction

Today, the ultimate solution in communication on histology is found in virtual microscopy. This technique enables digitizing complete tissue slides in high magnification, which are normally used to view with a conventional microscope, and store the information electronically on hard disk [3, 6]. Dedicated viewers can make the images visible, enabling a computer to become a functional microscope (see Fig. 5.1). The power of this technique is that all computers having access in a network, which can be as large as the Internet or Intranet, to the image server can produce the images, making distance to the image server unimportant, and thus forms a solid basis for communication. This concept can, of course, have major consequences for much of the work normally done with conventional microscopes. Here, we describe how virtual microscopy was implemented at Erasmus University Medical Center (Erasmus MC), the largest university hospital in the Netherlands, and what opportunities are expected from this technique in the future. The virtual microscope installed at Erasmus MC is a Hamamatsu Nanozoomer in combination with the included NDPserve, NDPview, and NDPscan software.

5.2
Steady Replacement of Microscopes

For clinical pathologists, a good-quality microscope is instrumental for accomplishing their daily task, although the virtual microscopic images are huge in their file size [7], ranging from 100 MB to over 2 GB, depending on the magnification, number of layers, and the area of tissue to scan. In addition, scanning takes its own time. However, despite these drawbacks, the virtual microscope, due to its advantages, is liable to take over more and more terrains in daily pathology. It starts with the use of these images in clinical work

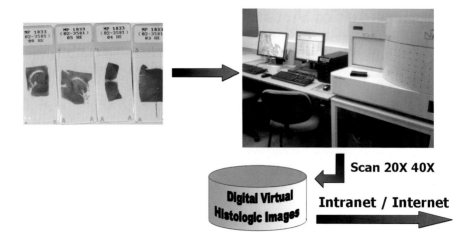

Fig. 5.1. Overview of how glass slides can be made visible in an Intranet–Internet environment by virtual microscopy: (**a**) the glass slide, (**b**) the virtual microscope, and (**c**) the storage disk for the images

discussions. Virtual microscopy can be used in every room with a computer connected to a beamer, whereas until now an especially equipped room was needed with a high-quality microscope with a video camera operated by the presenter, where the image is presented again with a beamer, or, as an alternative, a multiheaded microscope. As a consequence, the meeting can now take place in any room, preferably those where the PC is connected to the network containing the image server.

The bold ones even take the images on disk together with the viewer software to external meetings where the viewer is installed just before the presentation. The reaction on first use mostly is the appreciation of a much better contact with the audience during display of the images. In addition, the audience keeps an overview of the navigation through the slide, which enormously improves the transfer of knowledge.

5.3
Education

Knowing this, the next step, of course, is to introduce this technique in the medical education, where the keeping of many microscopes, which are mostly just up to quality because of budgetary limits, that all need to be maintained for a large amount of money forms perhaps even a stronger incentive. However, the idea that many students can try to access one particular image at the same time demands a proper setup, which needed to be tested on reaction time. Testing the facilities in close collaboration with Hamamatsu on response time in a classroom with 60 simulated students clearly showed that, on top of the already installed Intranet image server, a separate server dedicated to the education environment was needed. In addition, proper handling of requests and caching of the requested information were installed in the new version of NDPserve software on the dedicated image server. These changes caused the maximum response time to drop from over a minute to 10 s. In the Year 2007, the new curriculum started with full implementation of virtual microscopy instead of the microscopes. Figure 5.2 clearly illustrates the difference in the educational environment and the more easy interaction that can take place on the exchange of knowledge seeing the situation as it was in Fig. 5.2a in comparison with the actual situation Fig. 5.2b. A proper evaluation [2, 5] will have to wait until the student responses can be analyzed; however, the intermediate results of the surveys already look very promising.

5.4
Ring Trials

For reasons of quality assurance, ring trials are organized between the different pathology institutes in the Netherlands. In these ring trials, the glass slides, which need to be prepared in excess (one for every participating institute), are sent by regular mail from one institute to the other following a specific logistic order. This way, every institute can give their diagnosis on the cases sent around by regular mail. The outcome is then discussed in special meetings organized for this purpose. The virtual microscope can simplify these

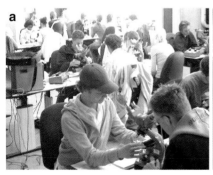
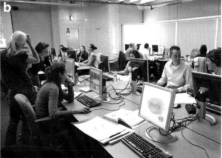

Fig. 5.2. Changed educational environment after implementation of virtual microscopy: (**a**) the environment with conventional microscopes and (**b**) the environment using virtual microscopy

logistics enormously by presenting this histology and case description on the Internet. In combination with a specialized application or simply starting with well-structured series of emails, the cases can be studied simultaneously from the same glass slide, without reproducing it from the original FFPE block.

5.5
Pilot for Implementation in Routine Pathology

Considering a routine pathology environment, virtual microscopy has a lot of advantages to offer over conventional microscopy. The logistics surrounding a glass slide can be simplified enormously, the risk of broken slides is decreased, and, most of all, the chance that a glass slide is missing once it has been scanned is almost zero – especially when a software is developed that automatically offers the image to the image server and puts the proper link in the laboratory management system. However, the yearly production of glass slides at a large pathology department can easily reach 200,000. In addition, a gradual rise in pathology cases is seen every year. Digitizing this large amount of glass slides for virtual microscopy typically demands up to 100 TB per year to store the images if only one layer is recorded. Different strategies can be applied to keep the budget for storage within bearable limits. It could be decided to make only part of the image archive dynamically available, whereas the rest could be available only on request. However, these costs are still enormous. It could even be decided to keep only the open cases on dynamic availability, and for up to 3 months after closure. During diagnosis, decisive simple images, representing only the part that is viewed, can be exported to the viewer and entered into the electronic patient file as a normal Jpeg image. The glass slide itself then forms the backup. However, it could be argued that a digital recording will keep the original color and contrast as seen when the glass slide is fresh, whereas the quality of glass slides diminishes over time.

Before such a giant step can be made, a pilot must be done to test the applicability of virtual microscopy in routine pathology, despite earlier reports on virtual microscopy in routine pathology [1, 4]. This pilot should cover a feasible amount for one virtual microscope and disk space. Before starting the pilot, the ideal image recording should be evaluated by the pathologists who will perform the pilot. In addition, the computer equipment of the pathologist should be optimized and could be improved by the use of two monitors instead of one. The advantage is that the pathology LIMS system can be operated on one while the image can be evaluated on the other. The outcome of this pilot will be decisive for further implementation. Both applications demand a viewer who gives the user the opportunity to use a set of carefully selected tools to perform the task needed.

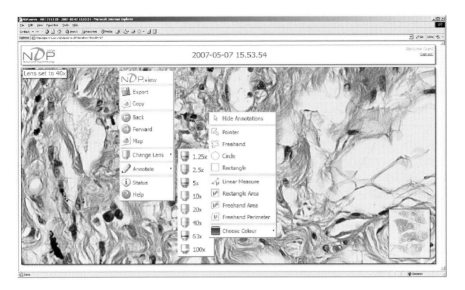

Fig. 5.3. Overview of options found in the NDP viewer

Therefore, a good viewer needs to be well equipped with such options reachable in an intuitive menu. An example of such a viewer is given in Fig. 5.3.

5.6
Privacy-Sensitive Network Environment

Many underestimate implementation of virtual microscopy in a hospital computer network. Such a network also has to govern patient data and therefore, in order to be protected by very strict rules, contains many high-quality firewalls. So, placing one image server in the hospital network to supply the Intranet of images is already a point of discussion. The IT department has a dedicated server room with servers all from the same brand and type, making operation and down time more easy to handle. Putting servers outside this server room is not allowed. However, the server was needed close to the virtual microscope to keep the scanning speed up to standard. This is typically required for the scanning process, which can only continue to the next slide when the collected data are all compressed and placed in a file on the image server after scanning. In addition, the sudden release of such an amount of data to be transported over the network to a server in the server room could easily overload the network and thereby seriously slow down others using the same network. This dataflow is therefore limited to a small gigabyte network, which is connected to the image server, which is, by way of official exception, connected to the Intranet of Erasmus MC.

The education environment is also shielded by a separate firewall from the hospital environment. So, exchange of images from the Intranet server to the education server is limited. However, permission has been obtained to view the images in the hospital environment for the teachers to prepare their educational material with the proper links and review the images at hand.

For the Intranet, a third image server was needed to operate in the demilitarized zone, resulting in the situation as represented in Fig. 5.4. However, for the Internet, the disk space is rather limited, due to the high costs involved for the user. Extra care must be taken to not release identifiable data with the image in, for instance, the filename. Most pathology slides are numbered with the pathology number, which is identifiable data and needs to be replaced by at least pseudonymization or even complete anonymization.

5.7
External Applications

5.7.1
Tissue Banking

Virtual microscopic images could be extremely helpful in the selection process of samples from tissue bank networks for medical research. Dynamic links stored in the database can make the images readily available. However,

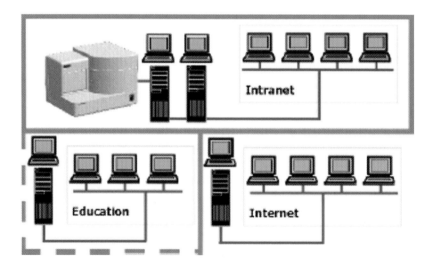

Fig. 5.4. Network environments in the different security levels that need to be serviced by virtual microscopy in an academic hospital

also due to the high costs for digital storage of the images, it is only feasible to use this technique for the known difficult pathology cases, as was already determined in the TuBaFrost project [6], where virtual microscopy was implemented in a central database application.

5.7.2
Multicenter Trials

For large trials that span more than one center, virtual microscopy can be a very helpful tool, especially when the diagnosis of all patients needs to be reviewed. For this purpose, the EORTC Tissue Bank Steering Committee developed a complete Web-based trial review system, which can make use of the links of virtual microscopic images stored on the Internet. This system was earlier described in detail [6], as was the use of virtual microscopy in trials [7].

5.7.3
Tissue Microarray Analysis

The virtual microscope produces images that are par excellence for the analysis of tissue microarrays (TMAs). The ability to have the overview of a complete array, coupled with the ability to view the arrays at high magnification, makes it the tool of choice, coupled with an analysis program for automated scoring and a database application keeping track of all the cores in a grid and of the results from different experiments on the same TMA. In one program, whole images of one TMA are stored for the different experiments together with the results, making the analysis far more comprehensive, but still orderly. Web-based TMA analyses are more and more asked for in the multicenter trial-related translational research, often using TMA techniques.

5.7.4
Histopathology Forum

Within the pathobiology workgroup of the OECI, a histopathology forum has been developed for the discussion of difficult, innovative, and interesting cases. Figure 5.5 shows a few of its pages in combination with virtual microscopy. This instrument fully supports one of the views of the OECI that new knowledge on cancer treatment should be spread faster over Europe, and, in addition, a form of gradual standardization can be reached, like in the earlier-described ring trials. Interestingly, the closed cases can form a repository of images for pathology students in their training.

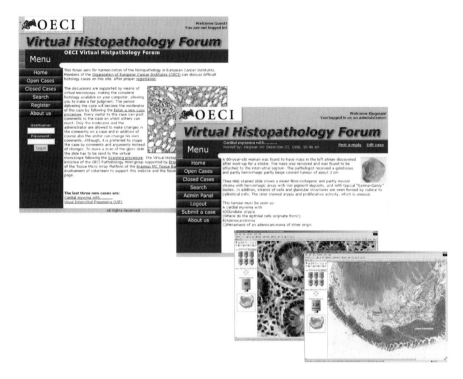

Fig. 5.5. Web-based OECI histopathology forum

5.8
Future Developments

Virtual microscopy will become the technique of choice over conventional microscopy when professional digital storage and backup systems become available for affordable prices. As there has been a steady drop in prices over the years since the introduction of the hard disk, it is expected that this point will be reached in the very near future. Another necessity for this technique to succeed is the compatibility of the now differently used formats in the available software. The best standard does not always win in a commercial environment. Especially, the dedicated software, e.g., TMA analysis, education, and image analyses must be able to cope with all the different formats. A prerequisite is that the dedicated software must, of course, stay affordable for the potential users.

In addition to the development, we have seen in educational material for medical students, depicted in Fig. 5.6, in time yet another development might be seen in this area – actual histology books with DVDs or Web-based solutions containing virtual microscopic images complete with annotations on the image for illustration.

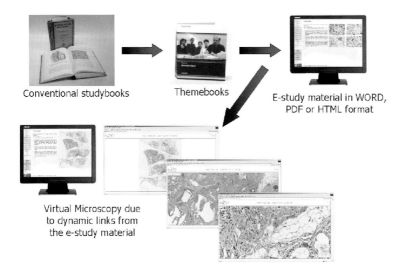

Fig. 5.6. Developments in study material

Another development is the increasing requests received from scientists to make virtual microscopic images: some for the reasons of comparing tissue slides or cells more directly, and others come for bringing virtual microscopy in image analysis to automated recognition of biological processes, where the overview and detail are both extremely important for the recognition process. In the far future, perhaps, automated recognition of virtual microscopic images can aid in the diagnostic process, where pathologists can work like pilots of an airplane by setting the process in motion and checking the final results.

5.9
Summary

- Implementation of virtual microscopy in an academic hospital
- Consequences of a privacy-sensitive network environment for implementation
- Intranet applications:
  - Pathology work discussions
  - Implementation of virtual microscopy in medical education
  - Developments in routine pathology (pilot)
- Internet:
  - Tissue banking
  - Multicenter trials
  - TMA analysis

– Ring trials
– Histopathology forum
■ Expected future developments for virtual microscopic applications
■ Medical research and virtual microscopy

Acknowledgments

Special thanks go to the staff of Hamamatsu for their kind cooperation in the implementation of the Nanozoomer in the different environments of Erasmus MC and their willingness to further adapt and develop the software on items we have encountered. In addition, all the patient cooperation I have had from the IT department made Erasmus MC virtual microscopy possible in all environments.

References

1. Dee FR (2006) Virtual microscopy for comparative pathology. Toxicol Pathol 34(7): 966–967
2. Goldberg HR, Dintzis R (2007) The positive impact of team-based virtual microscopy on student learning in physiology and histology. Adv Physiol Educ 31(3):261–265
3. Isabelle M, Teodorovic I, Oosterhuis JW, et al (2006) Tubafrost Consortium. Virtual microscopy in virtual tumor banking. Adv Exp Med Biol 587:75–86
4. Li X, Liu J, Xu H, et al (2007) A feasibility study of virtual slides in surgical pathology in China. Hum Pathol 38(12):1842–1848
5. Mills PC, Bradley AP, Woodall PF, Wildermoth M (2007) Teaching histology to first-year veterinary science students using virtual microscopy and traditional microscopy: a comparison of student responses. J Vet Med Educ 34(2):177–182
6. Teodorovic I, Isabelle M, Carbone A, et al (2006) TuBaFrost 6: virtual microscopy in virtual tumour banking. Eur J Cancer 42(18):3110–3116
7. Zwonitzer R, Kalinski T, Hofmann H, Roessner A, Bernarding J (2007) Digital pathology: DICOM-conform draft, testbed, and first results. Comput Methods Programs Biomed 87(3):181–188

Telepathology
in Veterinary Diagnostic Cytology

Paola Maiolino and Gionata De Vico

6.1
Background Information

Telepathology is a branch of telemedicine which includes teledermatology, teleophthalmology, teleradiology, and telesurgery. Telepathology has been described as the practice of pathology through visualization of images indirectly on a computer monitor rather than directly through a microscope and usually entails electronic transmission of the images to a remote site [21, 23]. Telepathology has several potential uses, such as remote primary diagnosis, expert consultation and consensus diagnosis, distant learning and teaching, research, and quality control. Telediagnosis is the most prominent application as it offers the advantage of exchanging histologic and cytologic images for diagnosis and consultation, especially at remote institutions where pathologists are not always able to be on-site and in cases in which a second opinion by an expert is required. Currently, when a difficult case is encountered during daily practice, this is carried out by sending the consultant the glass slides or paraffin blocks by courier or ordinary mail, but consultation often takes too long. Telepathology has been considered, in many human cases, an alternative approach.

It exists in two basic forms: static and dynamic. In static telepathology (also known as offline or store and forward), the microscope images are captured at one site and are then transmitted by email and viewed at a remote site. In dynamic telepathology, real-time images from a sophisticated robotic microscope are transmitted to a remote site. The remote operator has complete control of the field of view and magnification.

More recently, a variety of static, dynamic, and hybrid forms of telepathology permitting simultaneous transmission of real-time microscopy have been demonstrated. Such varied forms include videoconferencing and virtual microscopy.

6.2
Human and Veterinary Global Experience

The most widely published studies have considered surgical pathology specimens, including frozen and paraffin sections [3–6, 8, 15, 19, 20, 22, 24], while
few have considered telecytologic diagnosis [1, 2, 14, 17, 25, 26]. Telecytology
began with cervical–vaginal smears since when several workers have taken up
single organ systems like the breast, pancreas, and thyroid.

Raab et al. [17] examined the diagnostic accuracy of five cytotechnologists
who reviewed 50 cervical–vaginal smears using video monitoring and light
microscopy. In this study, the accuracy of telecytology was high but less than
that of light microscopy. Similar results were reported in the Ziol et al. [26] and
Alli et al. [1] studies on cervical–vaginal smears.

Subsequently, Yamashiro et al. [25] studied a large number of routine samples
(cervical smears and not) and reported a reasonably satisfactory concordance
rate between telecytodiagnosis and glass slide diagnosis for all samples (kappa
values were 0.92 for cervical smears and 0.81 for the other specimens) except for
biliary tract samples and fluids. The accuracy rate of telecytodiagnosis was high
and did not differ from that of conventional cytology.

Briscoe et al. [2] described a small telepathology trial on the fine-needle
aspiration cytology of the breast. The digital images and glass slides were
examined by three experienced cytopathologists. There was complete agreement between telepathology and glass slide diagnosis in 80–96% of cases,
although the pathologist with most experience in telepathology made the
smallest number of diagnostic errors. These results indicated that cytologic
diagnosis could be highly accurate using telepathology, although this depends
on the level of expertise of the pathologist in this technology.

Della Mea et al. [6] reported on a study of telepathology, using email transmission, 48 cases of fine-aspiration cytology of breast lesions, which were sent
from Udine to Trento, Italy. An agreement between local and remote cytodiagnoses was obtained in 43 cases (83.7%), whereas in four cases (8.3%) the
remote pathologist was unable to make a diagnosis as a result of insufficient
images and in one case as a result of an inadequate cytologic sample. These
results indicate that diagnosis of fine-aspiration cytology of breast lesions
could be made accurate by using static telepathology, although this depends
on image sampling and image quality.

Marchevsky et al. [14] described a small trial of static telepathology in pancreas cytology. They diagnosed 26 fine-needle aspirates of the pancreas simultaneously by telecytology and routine microscopy. The telecytology results were
more accurate than those obtained by microscopy.

Mairinger and Gschwendtner [13] expressed strong concerns about the
accuracy of telediagnosis on cytologic smears. They suggested that cytologic

diagnosis should be obtained by screening the entire slide and not by reviewing a small number of selected digitized images.

Unfortunately, few studies on telemedicine in animals are available to date and most regard teleradiology. Forlani [9] in a preliminary teleradiology study in dogs confirmed the usefulness and efficacy of this technique in veterinary diagnostic radiology. Papageorges and Tilley [16] described how teleradiology provides optimal medical services also in veterinary medicine.

Elsewhere we have reported a small trial of static telepathology on veterinary cytologic specimens [12]. This study was the first report of telediagnosis in veterinary medicine. Twenty cytology cases were examined by three pathologists, and a final consensus diagnosis was reached. Digital images, from each case, were captured and transmitted for telecytology consultation from Naples to Messina, Italy. The average time required to capture images was approximately 30 min per case. There was good agreement between the consensus diagnosis and the consultant's telediagnosis (85%) and between the consulting pathologist's telediagnosis and conventional glass slide diagnosis (100%).

Subsequently, we examined the diagnostic reproducibility of a series of veterinary cytologic cases (20) in which a diagnosis was made by three pathologists on both digital images and a light microscope. We found that intra- and interobserver diagnostic reproducibility for digital images and glass slides was fair to good even if interobserver diagnostic reproducibility was slightly higher for digital images than for glass slides. Pathologists were more likely to agree on the interpretation of digital images than on the interpretation of glass slides (P. Maiolino et al., unpublished data).

Recently, we demonstrated the usefulness and efficacy of telepathology by email also in veterinary diagnostic histopathology [11].

6.3
Guidelines for Preparation of Telecytologic Cases

A good cytologic smear is essential to obtain a high diagnostic yield; it must contain appropriate, representative, and well-preserved cells. Therefore, from each case, the most representative slide should be selected. For each case, at least six images should be captured (the more the better) – one image using a ×10 objective lens, one using a ×25, two using a ×40, and two using a ×100 objective lens. Low and intermediate magnification images are used to evaluate cellularity and cellular distribution (cluster and/or discrete cells) and cellular composition (inflammatory cells, epithelial cells, spindle cells, etc.), but also the appearance of crystals, foreign bodies, parasites, etc. High-magnification images are used to evaluate cellular details (such as nuclear-to-cytoplasm ratio, chromatin pattern, and presence of nuclear pleomorphism) and to identify and confirm the identity of organisms and inclusions. To capture the images, we recommend a digital still camera. A digital camera provides much higher resolution than a video camera, and it can be connected directly to a monitor. A personal computer with a 400 MHz processor and 128 MB of RAM, running a Microsoft operating system such as Windows 98 or most recent systems, is sufficient for telepathology. The images captured can be imported directly into Adobe Photoshop 5.0, stored in joint photographic experts group (JPEG) format (compression ration of 10:1), and transmitted with the patient's clinical history as email attachments through the Internet [12].

6.4
Limitations and Future Directions

Telepathology has the potential to become very important in diagnostics, but several problems have precluded its widespread use in daily practice [7]. Major impediments have included inappropriate selection of fields and insufficient image quality other than resistance from pathologists with negative preconceptions about the accuracy of this new technology [18].

Several factors may account for the higher accuracy in interpretation of digital images, as well as the selection of the field on the glass slide, technical factors (e.g., the inability to change the focal plane of the images), the ability of the person sending the images to identify and select the correct areas of the slide for transmission, and finally the experience of the pathologist.

Image selection depends especially on the experience of the pathologist in capturing and transmitting; image quality also depends on the computer hardware used. However, it is demonstrated that increased familiarity with telepathology combined with careful selection of the field on the glass slide for imaging improves these two factors.

Conventional glass slide diagnoses are generally obtained by screening the whole slide manually with a microscope. By contrast, cytologic telediagnoses are usually obtained by reviewing a small number of selected digitized images, considered to be representative of the case, on a computer monitor. The consultant pathologist selects the representative images of the case on the basis of his/her diagnosis and can steer the contributor pathologist toward the diagnosis. By contrast, the contributor should make his/her diagnosis on a restricted number of digital images of variable quality, and this may lead him/her toward diagnostic misinterpretation. In addition, digital images are easier and faster to examine.

Today, these problems can be overcome using dynamic (real-time) robotic telepathology. This system allows the consultant pathologist to control specimen orientation, field selection, and fine focus of the microscope. However, the cost of equipment and telecommunication is high, and there is no universal compatibility between several systems (static images are generally of higher quality and require lower bandwidths for transmission than dynamic images transmitted in real time).

6.5
Education and Training Opportunities Available

Pathology is a highly visual science. The inclusion of images of macroscopic and microscopic specimens in teaching, research, and electronic documents is fundamental. Those medical students, researchers, and technicians who hitherto used books, atlases, and slides can, today, access teaching material easily and at any time via the Internet. In addition, imaging, and especially digital imaging, is an important tool of pathology educators. Increasingly, they make use of digital presentations, as they are easy to prepare and inexpensive, can be stored on and disseminated by CD-ROM, and finally can be used also for lectures or presentations. Currently, there are numerous Web-based digital atlases for medical education (such as http://medlib.utah.edu/webpath/webpath/html, http://histology.nih.gov/, and http://www.webmicroscope.net/atlases/breast/brcatlas_start.asp), and there are many examples of the use of digital education (see the interactive Web site developed by Landman et al. [10] at the University of Pittsburgh Medical Center).

Potentially important applications of telepathology are:

- The documentation and teaching of medical procedures and techniques (such as complex surgical resection or organ fine-needle aspiration)
- Interdepartmental teaching, particularly for younger colleagues and especially in countries where pathology departments are situated at great distances from one another or where immediate transportation of specimens to a central pathology department is unsuitable and would be useful in facilitating the integration of international experts and in facilitating correlation between different subspecialties
- Quality assurance and quality control in pathology
- Proficiency testing in pathology

However, telediagnosis, above all expert consultations and primary remote diagnoses, remains the most prominent application, which is why a regionalization or even globalization of telepathology services can and should be expected. Telepathology is, therefore, not a substitute for conventional diagnostic procedures but a real improvement in the world of pathology.

6.6
Summary

- Telepathology is the process of diagnostic pathology performed on digital images viewed on a display screen rather than by conventional glass slide light microscopy.
- It has several potential uses, such as remote primary diagnosis, expert consultation and consensus diagnosis, distant learning and teaching, research, and quality control.
- Telediagnosis is the most prominent application, as it offers the advantage of exchanging histologic and cytologic images for diagnosis and consultation.
- Telepathology has the potential to become very important in diagnostics, but several problems have precluded its widespread use in daily practice: selection of fields and insufficient image quality other than resistance from pathologists with negative preconceptions about the accuracy of this new technology.
- Potentially important applications of telepathology are as follows: the documentation and teaching of medical procedures and techniques, interdepartmental teaching, quality assurance and quality control in pathology, and proficiency testing in pathology.

References

1. Alli PM, Ollayos CW, Thompson LD, et al (2001) Telecytology: intraobserver and interobserver reproducibility in the diagnosis of cervical–vaginal smears. Hum Pathol 32(12):1318–1322
2. Briscoe D, Adair CF, Thompson LD, et al (2000) Telecytologic diagnosis of breast fine needle aspiration biopsies. Intraobserver concordance. Acta Cytol 44(2):175–180
3. Cross SS, Burton JL, Dube AK, et al (2002) Offline telepathology diagnosis of colorectal polyps: a study of interobserver agreement and comparison with glass slide diagnoses. J Clin Pathol 55(4):305–308
4. Della Mea V (1997) Telediagnosis in pathology through the Internet. Telemed Virtual Real 2(7):75–76
5. Della Mea V, Puglisi F, Forti S, et al (1996) Telepathology through the Internet. J Telemed Telecare 2(Suppl 1):24–26
6. Della Mea V, Puglisi F, Bonzanini M, et al (1997) Fine-needle aspiration cytology of the breast: a preliminary report on telepathology through Internet multimedia electronic mail. Mod Pathol 10(6):636–641
7. Dervan PA, Wootton R (1998) Diagnostic telepathology. Histopathology 32(3):195–198
8. Eusebi V, Foschini L, Erde S, Rosai J (1997) Transcontinental consults in surgical pathology via the Internet. Hum Pathol 28(1):13–16
9. Forlani E (2006) Telemedicina, un caso pratico. Obiettivi e Documenti Veterinari 12:29–34
10. Landman A, Yagi Y, Gilbertson J, et al (2000) Prototype web-based continuing medical education using FlashPix images. Proc AMIA Symp 2000, pp 462–466

11. Maiolino P, Papparella S, Restucci B, De Vico G (2005) Telepathology in veterinary diagnostic histopathology. 23rd Meeting of the European Society of Veterinary Pathology, Naples
12. Maiolino P, Restucci B, Papparella S, De Vico G (2006) Evaluation of static telepathology in veterinary diagnostic cytology. Vet Clin Pathol 35:19–22
13. Mairinger T, Gschwendtner A (1997) Telecytology using preselected fields of view: the future of cytodiagnosis or a dead end? Am J Clin Pathol 107(5):620–621
14. Marchevsky AM, Nelson V, Martin SE, et al (2003) Telecytology of fine-needle aspiration biopsies of the pancreas: a study of well-differentiated adenocarcinoma and chronic pancreatitis with atypical epithelial repair changes. Diagn Cytopathol 28(3):147–152
15. Okada DH, Binder SW, Felten CL, Strauss JS, Marchevsky AM (1999) "Virtual microscopy" and the internet as telepathology consultation tools: diagnostic accuracy in evaluating melanocytic skin lesions. Am J Dermatopathol 21(6):525–531
16. Papageorges M, Tilley L (2001) Why telemedicine? Clin Tech Small Anim Pract 16(2): 90–94
17. Raab SS, Zaleski MS, Thomas PA, Niemann TH, Isacson C, Jensen CS (1996) Telecytology: diagnostic accuracy in cervical–vaginal smears. Am J Clin Pathol 105(5):599–603
18. Raab SS, Robinson RA, Snider TE, et al (1997) Telepathologic review: utility, diagnostic accuracy, and interobserver variability on a difficult case consultation service. Mod Pathol 10(6):630–635
19. Singson RP, Natarajan S, Greenson JK, Marchevsky AM (1999) Virtual microscopy and the Internet as telepathology consultation tools. A study of gastrointestinal biopsy specimens. Am J Clin Pathol 111(6):792–795
20. Strauss JS, Felten CL, Okada DH, Marchevsky AM (1999) Virtual microscopy and public-key cryptography for Internet telepathology. J Telemed Telecare 5(2):105–110
21. Weinstein RS (1986) Prospects for telepathology. Hum Pathol 17(5):433–434
22. Weinstein MH, Epstein JI (1997) Telepathology diagnosis of prostrate needle biopsies. Hum Pathol 28(1):22–29
23. Weinstein RS, Bloom KJ, Rozek LS (1987) Telepathology and the networking of pathology diagnostic services. Arch Pathol Lab Med 111(7):646–652
24. Weinstein LJ, Epstein JI, Edlow D, Westra WH (1997) Static image analysis of skin specimens: the application of telepathology to frozen section evaluation. Hum Pathol 28(1):30–35
25. Yamashiro K, Kawamura N, Matsubayashi S, et al (2004) Telecytology in Hokkaido Island, Japan: results of primary telecytodiagnosis of routine cases. Cytopathology 15(4):221–227
26. Ziol M, Vacher-Lavenu MC, Heudes D, et al (1999) Expert consultation for cervical carcinoma smears. Reliability of selected-field videomicroscopy. Anal Quant Cytol Histol 21(1):35–41

Use of Telepathology in Mohs Micrographic Surgery

Julie K. Karen, Klaus J. Busam, and Kishwer S. Nehal

7.1
Background

7.1.1
Mohs Micrographic Surgery

Mohs micrographic surgery is a specialized surgical and pathologic technique for the treatment of high-risk cutaneous neoplasms. Mohs surgery is a staged procedure that requires the dermatologic surgeon to function as both the surgeon and the pathologist. Small margins of normal-appearing tissue surrounding the clinically apparent tumor are excised in successive stages. The excised tissue is then processed via a fresh-frozen technique for immediate microscopic examination of the complete surgical margins. Excision proceeds until tumor-free surgical margins are achieved. The Mohs technique provides examination of 100% of the surgical margin and precise tumor mapping. Thus, Mohs surgery achieves high cure rates and is tissue sparing. Mohs surgery is ideally suited for the treatment of cutaneous neoplasms at high risk of recurrence, and for those occurring in areas of critical functional or cosmetic importance. Mohs surgery is most commonly employed in the management of high-risk basal cell carcinoma (BCC) and squamous cell carcinoma (SCC) [8]. The success of Mohs surgery depends on the ability of the surgeon to make quick but accurate conclusions about the presence or absence of tumor on frozen sections.

Mohs surgeons confront challenging intraoperative decisions about whether a structure of frozen sections is benign or malignant or the significance of inflammation. Tumors with unusual histology or findings of perineural invasion can also be challenging on frozen sections, and accurate assessment of these findings can impact overall patient management. These intraoperative challenges can be resolved in several ways. One option for the surgeon would be to remove an additional layer of tissue as a safeguard. However, unnecessary removal of even small amounts of additional tissue in critical areas can have significant cosmetic and/or functional implications for the patient. Alternatively, the surgeon could inaccurately conclude that a structure in question at the surgical margin is benign, when in fact it is malignant. In such a scenario, tumor extirpation would be incomplete, possibly leading to tumor recurrence.

Ideally, resolution of diagnostic challenges that arise during Mohs surgery would involve immediate consultation with a dermatopathologist. For Mohs surgeons practicing in close physical proximity to a dermatopathologist, intraoperative consultation can be achieved by simply bringing the slide in question to the dermatopathologist for review while the patient waits. However, physical distance or other barriers can preclude such immediate consultations. This is true, for example, for Mohs surgeons in private practice in areas remote from major universities or dermatopathology laboratories. When access to an on-site dermatopathologist is not feasible, the Mohs tissue layer in question can be sent for paraffin-embedded permanent sections. However, this approach delays wound reconstruction and inconveniences, the patient requiring an additional visit [11].

7.1.2
Telepathology

Telepathology is an emerging technology that uses telecommunications to transmit and visualize images, enabling remote pathology consultation and diagnosis. There are two major forms of image technology: static and dynamic telepathology. Static (store-and-forward) telepathology involves capture and electronic transmission of a few selected still digital images. The advantages of static telepathology include low equipment cost and ease of use. However, static telepathology can be limited by sampling error. Dynamic telepathology involves the transmission and visualization of real-time images. In its most complete form, the dynamic mode enables the remote pathologist to control all aspects of the microscope including magnification, focus, and slide navigation. Thus, dynamic telepathology closely mimics conventional light microscopy. Moreover, dynamic telepathology does not rely on image selection by another individual. The major disadvantage of dynamic telepathology relates to complex equipment needs and higher associated costs [3].

7.2
Telepathology in Dermatology

The feasibility of static telepathology for the diagnosis of cutaneous disease has been published [1, 4, 5, 12, 13, 15]. In a retrospective study involving frozen-section analysis of mainly nonmelanoma skin cancers by a surgical pathologist,

Weinstein et al. [15] demonstrated nearly 100% concordance of diagnosis and margin assessment between telepathology and glass slide microscopy. Similar results were attained by Dawson et al. [4]. Others have proven the feasibility of telepathology using paraffin-embedded permanent sections in the diagnosis of melanocytic lesions [5, 12] and other dermatologic entities [1, 13].

In a multiobserver store-and-forward study of 20 permanent-section skin specimens, Piccolo et al. [13] demonstrated high concordance between the telepathology and conventional histopathologic diagnosis. In this study, on average, 78 and 85% of diagnoses by telepathology and conventional light microscopy, respectively, were correct. A significant difference in accuracy was identified in only one case. Overall, despite slightly longer reading times, static telepathology by experienced dermatopathologists is feasible for the diagnosis of cutaneous diseases with frozen and permanent sections.

Morgan et al. [10] evaluated the feasibility of real-time, video-assisted telepathology by expert dermatopathologists. In this study, the two physicians agreed on greater than 85% of cases with telepathology compared with 96% concordance using conventional glass slide microscopy. A statistically significant difference was noted in the time required to render a diagnosis (19 s per case with a traditional two-headed microscope vs. 42 s per case with telepathology). However, while this difference might be important for a dermatopathologist whose practice is predominantly remote telepathology, it is unlikely to be significant in instances such as intraoperative consultations during Mohs surgery. In this study, discordance between telepathology and glass slide microscopy was attributed to limitations in equipment and telecommunications technology.

7.3
Telepathology in Mohs Micrographic Surgery

7.3.1
Feasibility

Nehal et al. [11] determined the feasibility of dynamic telepathology in Mohs surgery at Memorial Sloan–Kettering Cancer Center (MSKCC). In this pioneering study published in 2002, a dynamic telepathology system consisting of a microscope with a motorized stage and a video camera connected to a standard PC system was employed. The Mohs laboratory and remote-viewing site were connected through a local area network (LAN) and a wide area network (WAN). Using this system, a single glass slide was mounted on the automated microscope stage and completely scanned within minutes to create a virtual overview image of the glass slide. A single dermatopathologist located approximately 20 city blocks from the Mohs laboratory received the image on a large monitor running the dynamic telepathology software program. The software enabled control of slide navigation, objective change, and focus by both the local Mohs surgeon and the remote dermatopathologist.

A total of 110 skin specimens were selected for telepathology study (1) 50 permanent-section slides of BCCs and SCCs for pathologic diagnosis, (2) 40 frozen-section slides from Mohs surgery for the presence or absence of tumor, and (3) 20 frozen-section slides from Mohs surgery for intraoperative consultation. The same dermatopathologist later randomly reviewed all 110 glass slides by conventional light microscopy, and the diagnoses were compared. Concordance was 100% between telepathology and conventional light microscopy diagnoses. Both users rated the overall performance of the system as excellent. Image quality was deemed comparable to conventional light microscopy, and the system was simple to use. Initial shortcomings of the system included the inability to store multiple glass slide overview images for consecutive real-time viewing, as well as a relatively smaller field of view relative to conventional light microscopy. Occasional delays in remote robotic control and infrequent interruptions in the connection sometimes led to increased time spent evaluating the slides. This study proved the high accuracy of dynamic telepathology in the evaluation of fixed-tissue skin biopsies of nonmelanoma skin cancer and Mohs frozen sections for the excision of these tumors [11].

In 2004, Chandra et al. reported use of static telepathology for resolving challenges that arose during three difficult Mohs surgery cases. Image capture was achieved by direct application of a commercial digital camera lens to one microscope eyepiece. The captured image was then emailed to a pathologist. In these instances, immediate expert consultation permitted the surgeon to proceed with minimal delay and greater confidence [2]. Advantages of this system included ease of use and low equipment costs. However, potential sampling bias leading to inaccurate diagnosis remains a major limitation of static telepathology. Furthermore, there is concern over transmitting images via email due to potential security breach of confidential patient data [13].

7.3.2
Clinical Experience

In 2005, the MSKCC group described their clinical experience using dynamic telepathology for intraoperative consultation with a dermatopathologist during Mohs surgery. All relevant patient and tumor details were discussed with the consulting dermatopathologist, who was able to remotely control all components of the Mohs microscope [14]. During the 2-year period, a total of 61 intraoperative consultations were obtained during Mohs surgery. Reasons for requesting intraoperative consultations were divided into four main categories

(1) further defining tumor histology in 25 cases, (2) benign epithelial lesion vs. carcinoma in 22 cases, (3) basaloid follicular hamartoma vs. BCC in 10 cases, and (4) inflammation vs. inflamed residual tumor in 4 cases [14].

Questions pertaining to tumor histology typically arose when the tumor on Mohs frozen-tissue sections differed from the fixed-tissue biopsy diagnosis, when multiple tumor subtypes collided, or if the original diagnosis was not definitive. In addition, questions arose regarding the degree of differentiation of SCC or the presence or absence of perineural invasion. In addressing these important questions, telepathology consultation added important prognostic information. In 18 of the 22 cases in which the diagnostic dilemma was distinction of a benign epithelial lesion from a malignant tumor at the Mohs surgical margin, a definitive diagnosis of benign lesion or malignant tumor was rendered via telepathology, permitting appropriate further management without delay. In four cases, the diagnosis remained equivocal after consultation, necessitating an additional Mohs stage. In the ten cases in which the dilemma was distinction of BCC from basaloid follicular hamartoma, definitive diagnosis could not be rendered, consistent with the lack of diagnostic consensus on this entity. Finally, in the four cases in which the significance of inflammation was in question, telepathology consultation confirmed the absence of residual tumor, and the removal of additional tissue was avoided [14].

This study defined the scope of questions that arose during evaluation of Mohs frozen sections and established a role for intraoperative consultation with a dermatopathologist via dynamic telepathology in difficult cases. Overall, the use of dynamic telepathology directly enhanced patient care. In cases of definitive malignant findings at the surgical margin, further tissue removal was performed with confidence and without delay, achieving complete tumor clearance. In cases of definitive benign findings, the unnecessary removal of additional tissue was avoided. In equivocal cases, further excision was justified due to the uncertain biological nature of certain structures. In addition, dynamic telepathology permitted interdisciplinary education and collaboration, which benefited all participants [14]. The major limitation of widespread use of dynamic telepathology was equipment cost.

Recognizing dynamic telepathology as a convenient and attractive tool for intraoperative consultation during difficult Mohs cases, McKenna and Florell [9] sought to determine the feasibility of creating an inexpensive dynamic telepathology system. The authors devised a system based on the Internet and readily available consumer products (an off-the-shelf digital video camera and videoconferencing software). This system enabled a remote dermatopathologist to accurately interpret 20 fixed-tissue tumor slides and 20 Mohs frozen-section slides. In contrast to more sophisticated dynamic telepathology systems, this system did not allow robotic control by the remote dermatopathologist. However, a real-time audio link permitted concurrent verbal communication, enabling the dermatopathologist to guide slide navigation by the Mohs surgeon. With this improvised system, the authors achieved accurate and affordable dynamic telepathology.

7.3.3
Limitations

The limitations of telepathology in Mohs surgery are shared by other fields seeking to incorporate this technology into practice. These limitations relate to physician resources, technology, patient privacy, and cost. At the physician level, telepathology requires a dermatopathologist who has the confidence to participate in telepathology consultations. With initial use of telepathology, there is decreased confidence in making a diagnosis, which is overcome with increased experience [6]. Dynamic telepathology requires the referring Mohs surgeon and remote dermatopathologist to be available at the same time. An additional perceived problem relates to questions of the liability and responsibility of the consulting dermatopathologist. Technological limitations relate to the need for capture and transmission of digital images with high spatial and color resolutions [3, 7]. In addition, high-bandwidth communications are necessary to transmit high-quality images, especially if robotic control of the remote microscope is to be possible, as with dynamic telepathology. Patient privacy issues include questions surrounding the security and confidentiality of patient data transmitted on an open network [11, 14].

Finally, questions regarding cost–benefit analysis invariably surround discussions of using telepathology in Mohs surgery. Presently, high-quality dynamic telepathology systems are prohibitively expensive for a single user and overwhelm any cost–benefit analysis [7]. A particular problem with respect to Mohs surgery relates to the fact that the consultation with the dermatopathologist cannot be billed, as Mohs surgery reimbursement is predicated on the fact that the Mohs surgeon functions as both surgeon and pathologist [14].

7.4
Future Directions

In contrast to other fields where telemedicine has been met with great enthusiasm, to date, very few Mohs surgeons use telepathology. Technological advancements have helped to overcome some of the perceived problems regarding poor image quality and data security; however, problems relating to liability concerns and cost persist. Cost represents the major impediment to the adoption of sophisticated dynamic telepathology by Mohs surgeons. Innovative, low-cost Internet solutions, such as those described by McKenna and Florell [9], may have a role as more inexpensive alternatives. Technological innovation carries with it the promise of more feasible, affordable telepathology. The integration of telepathology by Mohs surgeons would permit accurate, convenient, and time-efficient assessment of challenging cases and, therefore, directly enhance patient care.

Utility of telepathology in Mohs surgery could be further enhanced by creating virtual libraries of Mohs cases, which would represent an invaluable educational resource for the training and self-assessment of current and future Mohs surgeons. Digitally stored images of tumors and their margins could be tagged to electronic medical records and/or could become a critical part in quality assurance. The availability of digital records would greatly facilitate the exchange of relevant information, if, for example, a patient develops a recurrence after prior Mohs surgery.

7.5
Summary

- Mohs micrographic surgery is a specialized surgical and pathologic technique for the treatment of high-risk cutaneous neoplasms.
- The Mohs technique provides examination of 100% of the surgical margin and precise tumor mapping and therefore achieves high cure rates and is tissue sparing.
- Mohs surgeons confront challenging intraoperative decisions about whether a structure on frozen sections is benign or malignant or the significance of inflammation.
- Resolution of diagnostic challenges that arise during Mohs surgery should ideally involve immediate consultation with a dermatopathologist; however, this is not always possible.
- Telepathology is an emerging technology that uses telecommunications to transmit and visualize images, enabling remote pathology consultation and diagnosis.
- The feasibility of telepathology for the diagnosis of cutaneous disease, and specifically in Mohs surgery, has been published.
- The limitations of Mohs surgery in telepathology relate to physician resources, technology, patient privacy, and cost.
- The integration of telepathology by Mohs surgeons would permit accurate, convenient, and time-efficient assessment of challenging cases and, therefore, directly enhance patient care.

References

1. Berman B, Elgart GW, Burdick AE (1997) Dermatopathology via a still-image telemedicine system: diagnostic concordance with direct microscopy. Telemed J 3:27–32
2. Chandra S, Elliott T, Vinciullo C (2004) Telepathology as an aid in Mohs micrographic surgery. Dermatol Surg 30:945–947
3. Cross SS, Dennis T, Start RD (2002) Telepathology: current status and future prospects in diagnostic histopathology. Histopathology 41:91–109
4. Dawson PJ, Johnson JG, Edgemon LJ, Brand CR, Halle E, Van Buskirk GF (2000) Outpatient frozen sections by telepathology in a Veterans Administration medical center. Hum Pathol 31:786–788
5. Della Mea V, Puglisi F, Forti S, et al (1997) Expert pathology consultation through the Internet: melanoma versus benign melanocytic tumors. J Telemed Telecare 3:17–19
6. Dunn B, Choi H, Almagro U, Recla D, Krupinski E, Weinstein R (1999) Routine surgical telepathology in the Department of Veterans Affairs: experience-related improvements in pathologist performance in 2200 cases. Telemed J 5:323–337
7. Krupinski EA, LeSueur B, Ellsworth L, et al (1999) Diagnostic accuracy and image quality using a digital camera for teledermatology. Telemed J 5:257–263
8. Martinez JC, Otley CC (2001) The management of melanoma and non-melanoma skin cancer: a review for the primary care physician. Mayo Clin Proc 76:1253–1265
9. McKenna JK, Florell SR (2007) Cot-effective dynamic telepathology in the Mohs surgery laboratory utilizing iChat AV videoconferencing software. Dermatol Surg 33:62–68
10. Morgan MB, Tannenbaum M, Smoller BR (2003) Telepathology in the diagnosis of routine dermatopathologic entities. Arch Dermatol 139:637–640
11. Nehal KS, Busam KJ, Halpern AC (2002) Use of dynamic telepathology in Mohs surgery: a feasibility study. Dermatol Surg 28:422–426
12. Okada DH, Binder SW, Felten CL, Strauss JS, Marchevsky AM (1999) "Virtual microscopy" and the Internet as telepathology consultation tolls: diagnostic accuracy in evaluating melanocytic skin lesions. Am J Dermatopathol 21:525–531
13. Piccolo D, Soyer HP, Burgdorf W, et al (2002) Concordance between telepathologic diagnosis and conventional histopathologic diagnosis. Arch Dermatol 138:53–58
14. Sukal SA, Busam KJ, Nehal KS (2005) Clinical application of dynamic telepathology in Mohs surgery. Dermatol Surg 31:1700–1703
15. Weinstein LJ, Epstein JI, Edlow D, Westra WH (1997) Static image analysis of skin specimens: the application of telepathology to frozen section evaluation. Hum Pathol 28:30–35

Combining Dynamic- and Static-Robotic Techniques for Real-Time Telepathology

Vincenzo Della Mea, Palmina Cataldi, Barbara Pertoldi, and Carlo A. Beltrami

8.1
Introduction

Telepathology is a subspecialty of telemedicine aimed at supporting the pathologist's practice by means of telematic tools. A number of different technical approaches have been developed, to solve different needs related to the practice of pathology at a distance, which is usually considered to include remote consultation [3, 19], intraoperative telediagnosis [16, 18, 23], quality control [9, 11, 14], distant education [1, 12], and remote image analysis [8, 13]. Some of these tasks need real-time communications and some do not, leading to different solutions.

One of the most regarded applications, with foreseeable success, is the intraoperative telediagnosis to be applied between small hospitals without pathology service and pathology services located elsewhere, for giving support to an isolated pathologist sometimes needing consultation, or even to completely transfer the diagnostic work in another Institute. This could lead either to better care or to expense reductions.

Intraoperative telediagnosis needs real-time methods for communication, because it is an urgent task, to be carried out as fast as possible; thus, it is not possible to adopt the so-called store-and-forward methods [2, 17], already proposed for remote consultation and quality control.

After the recent evolution due to the so-called digital slides (or WSI – whole slide imaging), store-and-forward telepathology received a strong push toward that technological advance, because it is still store and forward, but it makes the complete slide available at a remote observer. However, WSI cannot substitute real-time methods, as it is intrinsically asynchronous, although sometimes acquisition is very fast.

There are many technological ways to approach real-time telepathology, ranging from static- to dynamic-robotic solutions [16]. Real-time static systems are based on the delivery of still images in near real time; in dynamic systems, real-time video from the microscope is sent to the remote observer. No matter whether the system is static or dynamic, the microscope can be operated either directly by a physician or a technician or remotely by the observer. In the former case, the selection of fields is made necessary by the local operator, which can be guided vocally by the remote observer. In the latter case, a robotized microscope is used, together with a further software module for microscope operation; this way, a robotic – static or dynamic – telepathology system can be obtained. In particular, dynamic-robotic telepathology allows the specimen's observation in real time with the completely remote guide of the microscope, in a way similar to a normal session at the optical microscope.

Dynamic telepathology is usually implemented by means of videoconferencing or videoconferencing-like protocols, from which image characteristics are inherited; this means that images have a basic resolution of up to 352×288 pixels, which is currently regarded as too low for diagnosis, whereas static telepathology may adopt higher resolutions. On the other side, dynamic systems allow for an easy location of fields during diagnosis. This occurs in a way similar to the behavior of the microscope, whilst static systems can reach similar facilities by including a so-called slide-preview function, a sort of tiled low-magnification reconstruction of the whole specimen from which higher magnifications can be visualized.

In the recent times, videoconferencing protocols and systems have been developed for higher resolutions too, trying to match HD-ready and HD television specifications. However, such kind of image transmission needs a very large bandwidth, not always and reliably available.

The present work describes the diagnostic performance and the usability of a robotic telepathology system that incorporates dynamic as well as static features, with the possibility of choosing the most adequate modality at any time. The dynamic component can be used for locating fields and solving most of the diagnostic problems, while the static part can be used when the video image quality is not enough. The system has been tested on frozen section as well as on histologic and cytologic specimens, to investigate the range of its capabilities. In particular, attention has been drawn on the use of still images during a dynamic examination, to evaluate the added value given by such capability to a dynamic-robotic system.

8.2
Methods

Remote diagnosis has been carried out between the Institute of Pathology of the University of Udine, Italy, and the 60 km far Laboratory of Pathology of the City Hospital of Tolmezzo, Italy, located on the mountain area in the north of Udine. The Hospital of Tolmezzo has a surgical service, but it does not have a permanent pathology service, which is rather provided by an external consultant pathologist, coming twice a week from the Institute of Pathology of Udine. This of course allows only for scheduled surgery.

8.2.1
The Cases

A total of 184 histological and cytological cases were remotely analyzed using the telepathology system between the Laboratory of Pathology of Tolmezzo and the Institute of Pathology of Udine, during three phases: 60 frozen sections, 64 gastrointestinal biopsies, and 60 urinary smears, all unselected. Gastrointestinal biopsies and urinary smears were consecutively obtained from archives, while frozen sections were all the daily workload at the Hospital of Tolmezzo during the time of experimentation, and partly consecutively obtained from the archives. The cases from daily routine were previously diagnosed (including macroscopic handling and examination) by a different pathologist, in order not to give implications on surgical treatment. Macroexamination data were communicated to the remote pathologist when available in the archive records.

Gastrointestinal biopsy diagnoses were categorized as no lesions, inflammatory findings, benign lesions, and malignant lesions. The diagnoses of urinary smears were distinguished among insufficient material, not clinically significant (no lesions and inflammatory findings) and clinically significant (atypical issues and malignancy).

8.2.2
The Telepathology System

The system used for telediagnosis was a preliminary version of the Migra telepathology workstation (Olympus, Germany), which features both static and dynamic subsystems, in connection with a Sony 3CCD video camera (Fig. 8.1). The microscope was a Provis AX70 fully robotized microscope (Olympus, Japan), which has motor-driven stage, objectives, illumination, focus, and autofocus.

The Vision&Live dynamic subsystem (IAT, Switzerland) is based on the H320 videoconference protocol and uses up to three ISDN basic rate lines for transmission of real-time audio and video (equivalent to 384 kbit s^{-1} in the Euro-ISDN standard). It allows for selection of video sources, which are usually two, one linked at the microscope camera and the other at a desktop camera useful for videoconferencing between local and remote operator, together with an audio connection. The data channel of the system is used for remotely driving the robotic microscope, when available.

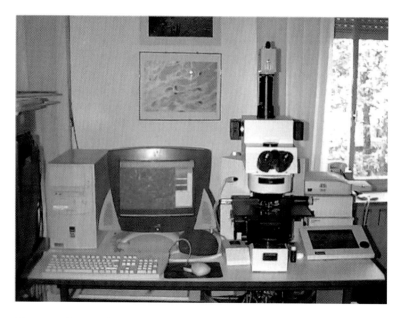

Fig. 8.1. The complete Olympus Migra telepathology system

The static subsystem, developed by Bildanalysis Systems (Sweden), is based on NetMeeting protocols (Microsoft, USA) and implements a shared workspace with cursor sharing and drawing and measure tools. Additional modules for case storage, management, and delivery through email are present. The static module uses another ISDN basic rate line (128 kbit s^{-1}) for image transmission.

The remote guide of the microscope stage occurs by means of a joystick; all other functions can be accessed through software buttons. Static and dynamic subsystems are fully integrated and receive the video input from the same source, although through two frame grabbers with different quality and resolution. The remote pathologist usually observes the glass slide by means of the dynamic module, navigating around it using the joystick and changing magnification and illumination when needed, thus seeing in the video monitor almost the same as if he/she were directly at the microscope. If the image quality is not satisfying, he/she can then request for a static image, which temporarily substitutes the video on the same monitor. The image can also be stored for further reference, saving also the coordinates of the acquisition.

8.2.3
Statistical Analysis

For each diagnostic session, the telediagnosis has been recorded, together with the time for microscopic diagnosis and the number and magnification of static images requested during diagnosis. The diagnosis at the microscope for each case has also been recorded, including the final diagnosis for frozen sections.

In the first phase, Tolmezzo was the referring telepathology workstation, while Udine was the consultant workstation, where the pathologist formulated the diagnosis by visualizing images on the monitor of the computer. In second and third phases, the roles were inverted, so Udine was the referring station and Tolmezzo the consultant station.

When communication errors or software problems occurred, a description of the problem has been recorded; comments on usability have been recorded too. Such reports have then been used by the developers to improve the system.

Diagnostic agreement has been described as percentage of corresponding traditional and telepathologic diagnoses; the precision of estimate for diagnostic accuracy has been given by means of approximate 95% confidence intervals (CIs), as suggested in [10]. We also calculated sensitivity, specificity, positive predictive value, and negative predictive value of the method for all cases, and separately for the three categories. Descriptive statistics of time and static images needed for each case has been given in the form of median and quartiles. Pearson correlation and linear regression have been applied to evaluate the dependence of static images and time.

8.3
Results

8.3.1
The Diagnoses

The evaluation of diagnostic accuracy in all cases showed an agreement of 94% (CI 92.2–96.8%). Diagnostic agreement for frozen sections was 100% (CI 97.5–100%). In gastrointestinal pathology, the agreement was 92.2% (CI 85.6–98.8%), with five discordant cases: two false negatives and three minor failures. The diagnoses of urinary smears had a total agreement of 90% (CI 82.4–97.6%), because six telepathological diagnoses of atypical smears were diagnosed as inflammatory findings or insufficient material at the microscope.

Table 8.1 shows sensitivity, specificity, positive predictive value, and negative predictive value of the method for all cases, and separately for the three categories.

8.3.2
The Time

The overall median time for the telediagnosis was 4′00″ (2′–5′45″). In frozen sections and gastrointestinal biopsies, the median time needed was

Table 8.1. Sensitivity, specificity, positive predictive value, and negative predictive value of the method

Cases	Sensitivity (%)	Specificity (%)	Positive predictive value (%)	Negative predictive value (%)
Frozen sections	100	100	100	100
Gastrointestinal pathology	67	100	100	97
Urinary cytology	100	100	100	100
Total	88	100	100	99

3′00″(2′00″–5′00″); finally, urinary cytology was diagnosed at distance in a median time of 4′30″ (3′00″–8′00″).

The highest time was recorded in a cytological case, with 23 min, which involved the transfer of four static images. In one occasion, software problems with the need to restart the computer led to 18 min for a frozen-section diagnosis.

8.3.3
The Static Images

An overall median number of 1 (0–2) static images was transferred for each case. In particular, frozen sections needed a median number of 1 (1–2.75) images, gastrointestinal biopsies 1 (0.25–2), and urinary cytology 1 (0–1). Overall, 58 cases (31%) have been diagnosed without the use of still images, while 71 cases (39%) needed only one image.

The overall time needed for transmission is slightly correlated to the number of static images transmitted ($r = 0.54$). Applying the linear regression analysis, this results in the following parameters:

Total time = 2′53″ + 1′22″ static images ($r^2 = 0.29$)

This could be interpreted as a part of the time being devoted to glass slide navigation by means of the dynamic subsystem, with a further part being devoted to static image transfer and analysis. This, in turn, fits in the diagnostic behavior patterns studied by Tsuchihashi et al. [26].

The relationship between failed cases and number of static images has also been investigated, discovering a slight and not significant increase in the average number of images in such cases. This can be due perhaps to some difficulties in the interpretation, in turn explainable to either the case difficulty or the glass slide quality.

Figure 8.2 shows the same field acquired through the dynamic (Fig. 8.2a) and static (Fig. 8.2b) subsystems; as it can be seen, the image quality is substantially different. Comments were transferred to developers, in order to enhance the

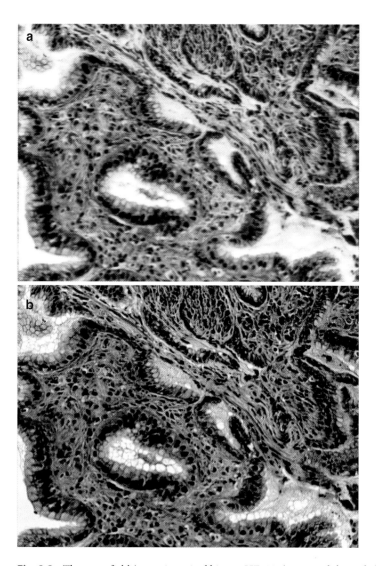

Fig. 8.2. The same field (gastrointestinal biopsy, HE, 20×) acquired through (**a**) the dynamic and (**b**) the static subsystems

usability of the system. As a result, a new version has been released, which also includes the slide preview and an alternative interaction system, based on the mouse. Occasional problems have been registered with ISDN lines, in particular when establishing the connection; this kind of problems should be taken into account particularly when dealing with frozen sections, because of the urgency needed for their diagnosis.

8.4
Discussion

The study involved three pathology fields; in the most important of these for its applicative possibilities, i.e., frozen sections, the system showed an extremely good behavior, from the point of views of diagnostic agreement as well as the time needed for diagnosis. The other two pathology areas, included in the study for completeness of evaluation, gave some additional information.

In gastrointestinal pathology, the agreement results are slightly better than those previously obtained using static telepathology [4]. In particular, two adenocarcinomas were diagnosed as chronic gastritis during the telepathologic session. In one case, the carcinoma was focal, with wider areas of severe dysplasia and microinvasion. In the second case, the carcinoma was present only in one of the fragments on the slide, while the others shown only the presence of chronic gastritis. Most probably, the discrepancy can be explained as follows: it is possible that, during the telepathologic session, the pathologist did not check the whole slide and missed the cancer.

A solution for this has been proposed as a support to the diagnostic activity in the telepathology software: a graphical mark of already visited areas on the specimen preview, which helps the pathologist in effectively examining the whole sample. Such a technical feature, present in other systems [6], is of help also in telecytological examinations and has been implemented in the last software release.

In cytology, the time needed for the diagnosis is higher than that needed in the other two fields, because the evaluation of single-cell morphology is the most crucial diagnostic step, and often material is spread around the glass slide. This effect has already been reported by others [22]. However, diagnostic discordance was mainly due to minor errors.

The experimentation carried out in this study allowed to evaluate the diagnostic accuracy of a dynamic-robotic telepathology workstation, as already made by others with similar results [7, 17, 21].

The studied system is particular, as it provides for both dynamic and static telepathologies, the latter thought as a way for overriding the classical resolution problems of videoconferencing-based dynamic systems. In fact, just a moderated number of still images are exchanged in many cases, giving a small time overhead but also an important possibility in respect to purely dynamic systems. The median time needed for a diagnosis is similar to the lowest times reported in the literature for real-time systems [21, 23], and lower than the results of static-robotic systems [6, 18], due to the locator functionality given by the real-time video capabilities. This, in our opinion, pushes toward integration between both modalities, to obtain both speed and, when necessary, the higher precision given by static images.

The adoption of telepathology should be preceded by an evaluation of savings that can eventually be reached in respect to more traditional solutions. However, when the aim is to give more support to an isolated pathologist, there are surely benefits on the diagnostic quality, which are difficult to be directly evaluated by means of economical analysis. However, real-time telepathology is needed only when such a support should be given in urgency and on demand, while, when decision can be delayed, WSI systems are more adequate nowadays.

Besides of this, the main problem that makes the adoption of telepathology as a mean for doing a completely remote diagnostic service difficult is the macroscopic sampling of the surgical specimen. In fact, although there are experiences where the surgeon is responsible for such a task [17, 20, 24], pathologists seem not to agree to let others do this important part of their work [15, 25]. In addition, legal aspects coming from the shared responsibility on the diagnosis should be studied.

The overall results allow us to consider the robotized telemicroscopy system as a helpful tool for delivering pathology services to isolated hospitals and, thus, to give a health-care service of the same quality as that given by central hospitals to otherwise underserved population. However, when real-time response is not needed, WSI may now be seen as the most appropriate solution.

8.5
Summary

- Features and limits of a dynamic telepathology system
- Advantages of hybrid systems
- A summary of experiences in histology, cytology, and frozen sections
- Hybrid systems and whole slide imaging

Acknowledgment

This chapter is partially derived from an article appeared in the journal *Analytical Cellular Pathology* [5].

References

1. Brebner EM, Brebner JA, Norman JN, Brown PA, Ruddick-Bracken H, Lanphear JH (1997) Intercontinental postmortem studies using interactive television. J Telemed Telecare 3:48–52
2. Della Mea V (1999) Store-and-forward telepathology. In: Hernandez B, Wootton R (eds) European telemedicine 1998/99. EHTO/RSM/Kensington, London
3. Della Mea V, Beltrami CA (1998) Telepathology applications of the Internet multimedia electronic mail. Med Inform 23:237–244
4. Della Mea V, Forti S, Puglisi F, et al (1996) Telepathology using Internet multimedia electronic mail: remote consultation on gastrointestinal pathology. J Telemed Telecare 2:28–34
5. Della Mea V, Cataldi P, Pertoldi B, Beltrami CA (2000) Combining dynamic and static robotic telepathology: a report on 184 consecutive cases of frozen sections, histology and cytology. Anal Cell Pathol 20:33–39
6. Demichelis F, Barbareschi M, Boi S, et al (2001) Robotic telepathology for intraoperative remote diagnosis using a still-imaging-based system. Am J Clin Pathol 116(5):744–752
7. Dunn BE, Almagro UA, Choi H, et al (1997) Dynamic-robotic telepathology: Department of Veterans Affairs feasibility study. Hum Pathol 28:8–12
8. Forti S, Eccher C, Visentin R, et al (1997) Distributed laboratory for remote image analysis in immunohistochemistry. J Telemed Telecare 3(Suppl 1):94
9. Haroske G, Meyer W, Kunze D, Böcking A (1998) Quality control measures for DNA image cytometry in a telepathology network. Adv Clin Pathol 2:143–145
10. Harper R, Reeves B (1999) Reporting of precision of estimates for diagnostic accuracy: a review. Br Med J 318:1322–1323
11. Kayser K, Kayser G (1999) Basic aspects of and recent developments in Telepathology in Europe, with specific emphasis on quality assurance. Anal Quant Cytol Histol 21:319–328
12. Klossa J, Cordier JC, Flandrin C, Got C, Hemet J (1998) A European de facto standard for image folders applied to telepathology and teaching. Int J Med Inform 48:207–216
13. Kunze KD, Böcking A, Haroske G, Kayser K, Meyer W, Oberholzer M (1998) Remote quantitation in the framework of telepathology. Adv Clin Pathol 2:141–143
14. Leong FJWM, Graham AK, Schwarzmann P, McGee JOD (1999) Controlled clinical trials of robotic interactive telepathology in the National External Quality Assurance Scheme. J Pathol 187(Suppl 1):5
15. Mairinger T, Netzer T, Schoner W, Gschwendter A (1998) Pathologists' attitudes to implementing telepathology. J Telemed Telecare 4:41–46
16. Nordrum I (1998) Real-time diagnoses in telepathology. Adv Clin Pathol 2:127–131
17. Nordrum I, Eide TJ (1995) Remote frozen section service in Norway. Arch Anat Cytol Pathol 43:253–256
18. Oberholzer M, Fischer HR, Christen H, et al (1995) Telepathology: frozen section diagnosis at a distance. Virch Arch 426:3–9
19. Perednia DA (1996) Reinventing telemedicine: store-and-forward applications. Telemed Telehealth Networks 2:15–18
20. Raab S, Robinson RA, Snider TE, et al (1997) Telepathologic review: utility, diagnostic accuracy, and interobserver variability on a difficult case consultation service. Mod Pathol 10:630–635
21. Schwarzmann P, Binder B, Klose R, Kaeser M (1998) Histkom – evaluation of active telepathology in fieldtests. Adv Clin Pathol 2:135–138

22. Schwarzmann P, Schenck U, Binder B, Schmid J (1998) Is todays telepathology equipment also appropriate for telecytology? A pilot study with pap and blood smears. Adv Clin Pathol 2:176–178
23. Shimosato Y, Yagi Y, Yamagishi K, et al (1992) Experience and present status of telepathology in the National Cancer Center Hospital, Tokyo. Zentralb Pathol 138:413–417
24. Szold A (2005) Seeing is believing: visualization systems in endoscopic surgery (video, HDTV, stereoscopy, and beyond). Surg Endosc 19(5):730–733
25. Tan YH, Preminger GM (2004) Advances in video and imaging in ureteroscopy. Urol Clin North Am 31(1):33–42
26. Tsuchihashi Y, Mazaki T, Nakasato K, et al (1999) The basic diagnostic approaches used in robotic still-image telepathology. J Telemed Telecare 5(Suppl 1):115–117

9

Telepathology in Iran

Afshin Abdirad and Siavash Ghaderi-Sohi

Pathology is one of the most important and most necessary services in every hospital. Nearly all health services need pathology diagnosis for perfect work. Expert pathologists are the most needed workers in this system. A pathologist may encounter difficult and complex cases during his/her routine practice that need consultation with an expert in the related field. Experienced pathologists are very valuable, and accessing to these persons is one of those favorite facilities that each coworker wishes to have. But finding a kind, interested expert pathologist to consult difficult problems is among the great expectations that each pathologist has in his/her life. Knocking next door and sitting down with an experienced colleague at a double-headed microscope whenever you want is not always possible for many pathologists, especially in developing countries. But it is not restricted to faraway centers. Pathology is a very vast specialty that includes many subspecialties. Practicing in all fields of pathology in a large general hospital is nearly impossible, and there is increasing need to consult cases with subspecialist experts in different fields. So, finding and consulting one of them may also be a problem encountered by pathologists who work in large academic centers in developing countries.

It is clear that the information and communication technologies (ICT) in the health sector could provide a better quality of life to the citizens and an easier job environment for physicians and other health-care workers. ICT can be used wherever it has a clear benefit, such as reaching remote populations, providing continuous training for doctors, and offering the tools for building a national health network.

While telecommunication systems are advancing rapidly in many parts of the world, those areas most in need of telemedicine services are likely to be the last to upgrade their telecommunications infrastructures.

Telepathology, a subspecialty of e-health, involves the use of telecommunication technology to transmit images to distant sites for purpose of communicating diagnostic information or for teaching. Recent advances in technology have greatly increased the feasibility of performing diagnosis by telepathology, but there are still significant obstacles to overcome.

In this chapter at first, we review briefly the state of telemedicine and telepathology in Middle East Arab countries, and then we discuss in more details about telepathology in Iran, the most populated country in this region.

9.1
Telepathology in Middle East

The use of telepathology is limited to a few centers in Arab countries of the Middle East that have about 270 millions populations [30]. The first documented experiment of static image telepathology in Kuwait and Arab world took place in 1999 [17]. Diagnostic microscopic images captured by a microscope-attached digital camera were selected by a pathologist in each case and sent with the clinical history to a second pathologist via email across the Internet. The diagnosis was sent back to the referring pathologist via email.

Amal cancer center in Amman, Jordan, has a telepathology section. This section consults with specialists at telepathology centers at Rotterdam and Leiden University in the Netherlands (2002) [33].

e-MedSoft.com is a leading application service provider (ASP) of comprehensive health-care information solution, has a Medreach™ telemedicine and a Medmicroscopy™ telepathology application that is selected by Medunet (a Saudi Arabic company). Medunet is a partnership between the Sultan Bin Abdulaziz Al-Saud Foundation and IMED Link, Inc., a USA-based provider of telemedicine services, medical and educational content development, advanced software design, and innovative network solutions to the Kingdom of Saudi Arabia. Medunet currently is a leading e-health service provider in Kingdom of Saudi Arabia. Through its satellite, microwave, and wireless networks, Medunet provides real-time classes, symposia, and distance grand rounds with leading US health-care institutions. Medunet has agreements with George Mason University School of Nursing to provide nursing education classes and with Columbia Presbyterian Medical Center and others for telemedicine services. Medunet also provides Internet and email services to over 10,000 physicians in the Kingdom of Saudi Arabia and recently launched its Web portal, Healthnet (http://www.health.net.sa), to focus on regional health-care issues [22].

Massachusetts General Hospital has spun off a subsidiary, American Telemedicine International (ATI) in recent years to provide telemedicine services to some centers in Riyadh. Telepathology is possible in this service [18].

In another collaboration project between the medical schools of Aberdeen University and the UAE University, telepathology teaching was conducted and evaluated. All students participating in the telepathology teaching sessions exceeded the minimum acceptable score of 60 in a multiple-choice examination [7].

A telemedicine service is also linked Apollo group of hospitals in India (New Delhi and Hyderabad) to Muscat, Oman. This service offers telepathology and teleradiology. This modality is also extended for conducting continuing medical education program for physicians in Oman [2].

9.2
Telepathology in Iran

In Iran up to October 2007, all published works in this field are confined to two studies. The first has evaluated the telepathology consultation of 161 cases through the use of iPath server of Basel University [1] and the second work has compared teleconsultation results of some cases from Iran and Germany [25]. The routine use of telepathology in the official Institutes in Iran is confined to telepathology service in Cancer Institute of Tehran Medical University. This center was active for 3 years (2001–2003) for teleconsultation of problematic cases referred to this center using iPath telepathology server of Basel University. There were no other special center, network, compatible software, and equipments for routine use of telepathology in almost all pathology institutes until recently. The pathologists who trained in Iran have little familiarity with telepathology. Therefore, we can say that despite the increasing development of telepathology and tendency for using it in routine work, it is in the beginning of its long way in this country.

We can look at telepathology in its four aspects in Iran:

1. Teleconsultation
2. Remote primary diagnosis
3. Remote education
4. Quality assurance programs

9.2.1
Teleconsultation in Iran

Consultation to reach an expert idea or second opinion is well known and is of value in pathology. UICC has estimated that a pathologist needs to consult 10–20% of cancer cases in his/her routine work [14]. This can make many problems for a pathologist. Sending glass slides or paraffin blocks by mail or courier for experts in the field is a time-consuming way, especially in critical specimens for pathologists working alone in distant hospitals with no facilities for consultation. Besides, the probability of loss and damage are always present [27]. Today, telepathology in two forms of static and dynamic seems to be the basic solution for this major problem. Teleconsultation in Iran could have many benefits regarding the ecological and economical and centralization of the specialty and equipments in a few centers, especially in Tehran.

According to the Iran national portal of statistics, about 40% of pathologists of ministry of health are only in two provinces of Iran, which have about 27% of the total population [28]. On the other hand, almost all expert pathologists are centralized in Tehran and a few of them in some other important provinces such as Shiraz, Mashhad, and Isfahan. Under the provision of health ministry, all new pathologists (specialists) should spend first few years of their career in remote areas, mostly alone without any opportunity to reach experts. Therefore, there is a complex status here in Iran:

1. A new trained pathologist, who is in more need of consultation, has the least chance to access.
2. Centralization of all expert pathologists in one or two large cities limits their accessibility.
3. Long distance between the province centers (at least 300 km), especially in the south of Iran, confines routine consultation.

These problems make consultation to be a very time-consuming and expensive affair, which causes delay in diagnosis with coast effect for patient and pathologist and often with the least advantage for the patient.

Regarding these limitations, teleconsultation could be a good remedy. Static and dynamic telepathology can be used for this purpose. However, expensive equipment, special software, and high bandwidth that are necessary for dynamic telepathology make it unavailable in many areas of Iran. The static telepathology service is relatively cheap and easy to set up, and all it needs are a microscope, a digital camera, and a line with medium-to-high bandwidth to access the Internet. All of these are accessible in nearly all pathology centers in Iran. The only limitation of the static telepathology is field selection, which causes approximately 15% low accuracy in comparison to dynamic one [8, 15, 31]. But it is acceptable in the presence of the inappropriate and ineffective system of consultation, which is now prevalent in Iran. There are also isolated reports of 95–100% accuracy in static telepathology [9], and it has been proved in many studies that this problem could be significantly improved by training pathologists and setting up well-defined protocols for sampling of different specimens [10, 24]. It is also clear that gradually this problem will decrease with increasing experience [16]. Thus, it seems that education and clear guidelines are essential before starting static telepathologic network. By installing regional software to connect small rural centers to referral ones, noticeable time and money can be saved with more efficient output. This is a duty that is in process now (see the next sections).

9.2.2
Remote Primary Diagnosis in Iran

This is a form of telepathology that is used in centers without on-site pathologist and has been used to provide frozen-section service in small rural hospitals. It is also used for teleconsultation in regard of its higher accuracy. This is performed through dynamic telepathology and needs motorized stage microscope, digital or charge-coupled device (CCD) video camera, special software, high-bandwidth network connection, and high-resolution monitors. The price to set up this system fluctuates in the range of $20,000–$100,000 [23].

Reasons that make dynamic telepathology inefficient in Iran include:

1. Absence of small center in rural area to perform surgeries, which may need intraoperative pathologic consultation.
2. The high price of equipments in this field makes it not applicable. Therefore, it would be wise to refer patients to centers with inside pathologist.
3. Telepathology is in the beginning of its way in Iran, and many authorities recommend that it should begin with static mode at first and gradually with achieving experience and getting more familiarity; it could be upgraded according to special demands to dynamic mode [23].

Therefore, we could say that remote primary diagnosis with dynamic intraoperative teleconsultation is not a necessity in contrast with teleconsultation with static mode in Iran.

9.2.3
Remote Education in Iran

More than 14 universities are training pathologists in Iran. However, regarding the points in previous sections about the uneven distribution of facilities, many complex surgeries are not performed in most of these centers, and the new procedures are confined to a few centers in large cities. For example, many of these centers have no IHC, molecular pathology and genetic facilities, electron microscopy, or transplantation ward or many other special sections. It leads to decrease of the numbers of specimens in pathology laboratories and limits them to a few routine repetitive cases without educational benefits for trainers.

Tele-education is already widely used and popular among pathology students in Iran. They have access to online recourses and databases with a series of images in different fields of pathology. This form of tele-education is popular worldwide and is also accessible in all centers in Iran. But it is not specific and not designed according to the special need of different geographical regions.

Regarding the centralization of most specialty and expertise in Tehran and few large cities of Iran, it seems that designing and planning a telepathology system with access to important surgical and clinical cases or the prime centers according to the prevalence and importance of the problem in Iran can be more useful for pathology residents. It should make accessibility to special wards; their tasks, protocols, and approaches to the patients; and also their important cases through an e-learning program and through a database for important cases. It needs coordination of universities, ministry of health, and allocation of resources, which seem to be a difficult task, but it would have many benefits.

Until accomplishment of this telepathology service, it is possible to establish virtual slides and microscopy in major centers, to prepare a good database of cases, which can be used for educational purposes. Virtual telepathology is almost completely in disguise in Iran and among pathologist. In this technology, a conventionally prepared glass slide is placed on a motorized stage of a microscope with capacity of automatic focusing. The slide is scanned completely and consequently using all object lens, and then these images are integrated to produce a single large image file [3, 29]. This file can then be viewed in a computer in each location. All the things it needs are a microscope with automatic motorized stage and a digital camera in addition to appropriate hard-disk space and software [3], which is not so expensive. We think the first step is to equip the referral centers in Iran with this technology to prepare a digital database of important cases, which will never change in appearance as long as the data integrity is maintained. It needs some education about virtual telepathology, e.g., through some workshops. Also, main centers are better to have virtual pathology instruments.

An important aspect of tele-education, which could be used in Iran to overcome cultural obstacles, is in the field of postmortem study and autopsy. There is not a full active center of autopsy in Iran. Some centers perform limited sporadic autopsies, which are not sufficient to have educational benefits. Therefore, investing capital to perform videoconferencing link between these centers is not wisely. Instead, it would be better to prepare some videoconferencing links with other foreign active centers. For example, we could point to United Arab Emirates University, which established a videoconferencing link with Aberdeen University of UK in 1997 [6] to provide the opportunity of acquaintance with this important field of pathology for its students despite the cultural limitations.

We can expand our viewpoint and establish a videoconference link between referral centers and others to cover the CPC conferences, which would have much educational benefit. These CPC conferences are disposed just in few centers, and many of our pathology and other specialty students have no chance of participating in these valuable sessions. For example, we can mention to the tumor board of the regional hospital of Lorrach (Germany), which has been running on iPath since 2001. The cases are preloaded before the conference, and during the tumor board the important points of contributors are added to the case [5].

We think that tele-education in the form of virtual pathology and videoconferencing link between centers is not just a desire in Iran, and we have prepared its preliminaries that we will describe at the end of this chapter.

9.2.4
Quality Assurance Programs in Iran

Quality management is an important aspect of all laboratory procedures. It is a special field in pathology. Quality control in the field of clinical pathology already performs to some extent in Iran; however, it should be improved to be perfect in the future. But it is not a routine task in surgical pathology. There are many reasons such as the absence of special organization in charge of this act.

External quality assessment (EQA) through the telepathology services in the field of surgical pathology is almost a new aspect in telepathology. It has many benefits, such as all participants study exactly the same specimens, a little time is needed to perform and evaluate the answers, and finally it is a useful way of distributing materials of small biopsies that are too small for replicate sections [26]. This type of EQA is already widely used in the UK [26].

Regarding the improper quality programs in Iran, it seems that designing a unique system, which can be accessible in all institutes and laboratories, can help in increasing the quality of these programs. However, this is just a hypothesis, and it is not the first object of telepathology in Iran. It should be set up first, and, gradually, while all pathologists adopt it as a useful system in their work, other aspects can also be noticed.

9.3
Problems

There are universal problems in different forms of telepathology, such as high cost, ineffective software, lack of compatibility between telepathology systems, poor network communication, quality issues such as image quality, and some legal issues that are not the scope of this chapter to discuss [32]. We have the regional problems in addition, which should be resolved prior to any effort of setting up an effective telepathology system in Iran.

The first and most important problem is unfamiliarity of almost all pathologists with telepathology, its benefits, and potential flaw. Although it has passed its infancy in many countries, it is in the beginning of the way in our country. Therefore, many of the pathologists have no familiarity with it and a few who know it do not have any tendency to use it in their routine work because of not availability of equipments, unfamiliarity of other pathologists with it, and fear of potential legal problems. We have no documented study about the skill of our pathologists in using telepathology systems in their work or their attitudes about it. However, as we see in our practical daily works, many of them have no skill to manage their cases through telepathology services and even the skill of capturing digital images of slides. This is not just our problem. A study in UK demonstrated that, despite the availability of digital imaging equipment, the levels of usage are surprisingly low and few pathologists had access training in digital image technology [11]. It seems that at least integrating the telepathology consultation course in pathology training programs can enable the new trained pathologist to get acquainted with the basic principle of telepathology. Meanwhile, setting up the telepathology service compatible with our regional characteristic and managing continuous courses of education for postgraduate pathologists could be effective in changing their opinion about use of telepathology in their routine works and taking into account the benefits of replacing conventional pathology by virtual pathology.

The cost of some type of telepathology systems such as dynamic mode, which have high price regarding the limited budget of our health system, is another problem and it is not cost effective. Therefore, we have to exclude the dynamic telepathology from our future project and focus on static telepathology and virtual pathology and change the conception of our pathologist about the telepathology.

9.4
What Have Been Done?

As mentioned earlier, we managed a teleconsultation unit for 3 years (2001–2003) in Cancer Institute of Tehran Medical University, with iPath server.

We evaluated our cases, and the results were published in *Diagnostic Pathology Journal* [1]. Out of 161 cases consulted, in 55% a definite final diagnosis was achieved. In 26% of the cases, a recommendation for complementary procedure was made and finally in 19% no definite diagnosis had been made. We found that the rate of achieving final diagnosis was higher in pathology cases than in cytology. Our finding was very far from other similar studies in achieving definite final diagnosis in 90–95% [4, 12, 13]. Most of these cases are problematic ones, which many studies stated that are not suitable for telepathologic consultation, because in many of them paraffin blocks are needed for more specific evaluation [10, 19], as it occurs in 26% of our cases. We proposed to design a software compatible with Iran network characteristics to connect small rural centers to referral ones, for performing the present numerous requests for consultation and subsequently saving time and money.

After the publication of our study, we intended to create a national server for telepathology to connect different centers in Iran. We preferred to take the advantage of experiences of one of the most popular server in telepathology in the world, i.e., iPath server, instead of designing completely new software, which could make a considerable delay. This was done by great helps of Kurt Brauchli from Switzerland. He also kindly gave us server in Basel University and helped us a lot to set up our telepathology site (http://www.telepathology.ir). iPath is a flexible telepathology system with many modality and potential functions. iPath has three choices for users (1) registering with an existing discussion group, (2) starting your own group, and (3) installing your own iPath server. We select the third option in which we have the complete freedom on what we want to do with our system. The system is developed under Linux Apache/PHP and Postgres–SQL and also running under windows with IIS and MySQL databases, Microsoft SQL server, or Oracle [20]. This type has been used till now by several centers such as West African Doctors Network, Inland Northwest Health Service for the Spokane district, and breast carcinoma field studies in Dresden, Germany [5]. With the help of Basel University, we establish our iPath server, Iranian Telepathology Center, (http://www.telepathology.ir) in Cancer Research Center of Tehran Medical University in May 2007 (Fig. 9.1). It was opened formally at the

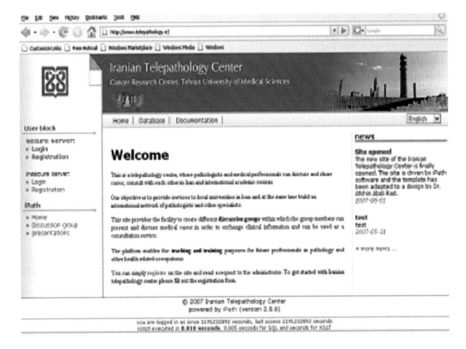

Fig. 9.1. The first page of Iranian Telepathology Center (http://www.telepathology.ir)

end of November 2007. It is completely like original iPath server with the rational database, which could collect all data transferring between the participants. It has many options for different uses. We can make different groups in which different cases could be present with their own data composed of the clinical data, radiographies, images, the question about it, and opportunity to see different comments about the present case. A candidate for a group should first register an account for the server and then contact with his desired group administrator for group membership. It has the possibility of using in dynamic mode by telemicroscopy option, and it has free downloadable software of microscope controller. In this mode, the expert can choose to add a selection of the pictures that the expert thinks should be added to the presented case, or it can be used for distance primary diagnosis, e.g., in frozen sections. It also has the option of remote presentation of a case, with possibility of simultaneous remote control and use of the chat box to comment your slides or shared pointer to point to interesting areas. It also has the possibility of combining a distributed presentation with an audio stream for transmitting the voice of the presenter. With combination of this option and the chat opportunity, we can also manage interdisciplinary conferences. We also add to this server the possibility of typing Farsi for Persian users. It has many other potential options, which are not in the scope of this chapter. Interested persons can see the iPath manual [21].

As we see, with this predesigned excellent software, we could manage all our objects in telepathology in Iran. We are going to introduce it to all pathologists by managing some workshops around the country. We wish to make different groups of special area of pathology with participation of experts in each field as administrator to manage our consultation requests from all parts of the country. Publishing educational pamphlet and presentation of weekly tumor board of cancer institute are also in progress.

Telecase is the other site of telepathology in Iran. Telecases.com is presented and launched for the first time on 7 July 2006 during the 8th Congress on Telepathology and Virtual Microscopy (Budapest, Hungary). It is backed, financially and academically, by Dental Research Center and Department of Oral and Maxillofacial Pathology at Tehran University of Medical Sciences, and it is dedicated to oral pathology. This is active in teleconsultation and has none of the iPath options. Although it is working for more than 1 year (from September 2006), it seems that it is not so popular among pathologists and oral pathologists. This emphasizes changing the pathologist's viewpoint of telepathology and its benefits, before any attempt to construct telepathology services in Iran. Achieving new hardware is not the main problem in developing countries, but changing minds to use new facilities is the main obstacle.

9.5
Summary

- Telepathology, a subspecialty of e-health, involves the use of telecommunication technology to transmit images to distant sites.
- The use of telepathology is limited to a few centers in Arab countries of the Middle East.
- We can look at telepathology in its four aspects in Iran: teleconsultation, remote primary diagnosis, remote education, and quality assurance programs.
- There are universal problems in different forms of telepathology, such as high cost, ineffective software, lack of compatibility between telepathology systems, poor network communication, quality issues such as image quality, and some legal issues.
- To create a national server for telepathology to connect different centers in Iran, we took advantage of one of the most popular server in telepathology in the world, iPath server, which is a flexible telepathology system with many modality and potential functions.

References

1. Abdirad A, Sarrafpour B, Ghaderi-Sohi S (2006) Static telepathology in cancer Institute of Tehran University: report of the first academic experience in Iran. Diagn Pathol (serial on the Internet) 1:33. DOI 10.1186/1746-1596-1-33 (cited October 04, 2007). Available from http://www.diagnosticpathology.org/content/1/1/33
2. AMC to launch telemedicine facility. The Oman Time. August 07, 2007. Available from http://www.timesofoman.com/archives_details.asp?detail=8987
3. Bacus Laboratories, Inc., Lombard: virtual microscopy. August 07, 2008. Available from http://www.bacuslabs.com/blog/general/VirtualMicroscopy.html
4. Brauchli K, Jagilly R, Oberli H, et al (2004) Telepathology on the Solomon Islands – two years' experience with a hybrid Web- and email-based telepathology system. J Telemed Telecare 10(Suppl 1):14–17
5. Brauchli K, Oberli H, Hurwitz N, et al (2004) Diagnostic telepathology: long-term experience of a single institution. Virch Arch 444:403–409
6. Brebner EM, Brebner JA, Norman JN, Brown PAJ, Ruddick-Bracken H, Lanphear JH (1997) A pilot study in medical education using interactive television. J Telemed Telecare 3(Suppl 1):10–12
7. Brebner EM, Brebner JA, Norman JN, Brown PAJ, Ruddick-Bracken H, Lanphear JH (1997) Intercontinental postmortem studies using interactive television. J Telemed Telecare 3:48–52
8. Callas PW, Leslie KO, Mattia AR, et al (1997) Diagnostic accuracy of a rural live video telepathology system. Am J Surg Pathol 21:812–819
9. Cross SS, Burton JL, Dube AK, et al (2002) Offline telepathology diagnosis of colorectal polyps: a study of interobserver agreement and comparison with glass slide diagnosis. J Clin Pathol 55:305–308

10. Cross SS, Dennis T, Start RD (2002) Telepathology: current status and future prospects in diagnostic histopathology. Histopathology 41:91–109

11. Dennis T, Start RD, Cross SS (2005) The use of digital imaging, video conferencing, and telepathology in histopathology: a national survey. J Clin Pathol 58:254–258

12. Desai S, Patil R, Chinoy R, et al (2004) Experience with telepathology at a tertiary cancer centre and a rural cancer hospital. Natl Med J India 17(1):17–19

13. Desai S, Patil R, Kothari A, et al (2004) Static telepathology consultation service between Tata Memorial Centre, Mumbai and Nargis Dutt Memorial Charitable Hospital, Barshi, Solapur, Maharashtra: an analysis of the first 100 cases. Indian J Pathol Microbiol 47(4): 480–485

14. Dietel M, Nguyen-Dobinsky TN, Hufnagl P (2000) The UICC telepathology consultation center. International Union against Cancer. A global approach to improving consultation for pathologists in cancer diagnosis. Cancer 89(1):187–191

15. Dunn BE, Choi H, Almagro UA (1999) Routine surgical telepathology in the department of Veterans affairs. Experience related improvements in pathologists performance in 2200 cases. Telemed J 5:323–332

16. Dunn BE, Choi H, Almagro UA, Recla DL, Krupinski EA, Weinstein RS (1999) Routine surgical telepathology in the Department of Veterans Affairs: experience-related improvements in pathologist performance in 2200 cases. Telemed J 5:323–337

17. Francis IM, Junaid TA, Dajani YF (1999) Static image telepathology in routine surgical pathology diagnosis: a report on the first experience in the Arab world from Kuwait. Med Princ Pract 8(4):255–265

18. Goodspeed L (1994) Telemedicine links Riyadh to MGH. Available from http://focus.hms.harvard.edu/1994/July22_1994/Technology.html

19. Halliday BE, Bhattacharyya AK, Graham AR, et al (1997) Diagnostic accuracy of an international static-imaging telepathology consultation service. Hum Pathol 28:17–21

20. History of iPath. August 07, 2008. Available from http://www.fsm.ac.fj/pws/Telepath/History%20of%20iPath.doc

21. iPath Manual. August 07, 2008. Available from http://ipath.ch/site/manual

22. Jacksonville Beach FL (2001) e-MedSoft.com announces agreement with MeduNet to supply telemedicine & telepathology solutions to Saudi Arabia and the Middle East. Trestle Corporation. Available from http://trestlecorp.com/press_archiveDetail.asp?ID=4

23. La Rosa FG (2008) Store and forward telepathology. Telepathology Consultant, P.C., Lakewood. August 07, 2008. Available from http://www.telepathology.com/articles/telepathology/Store&Forward%20TP.doc

24. Mea VD, Cataldi P, Boi S, Finato N, Palma PD, Beltrami CA (1999) Image sampling in static telepathology for frozen section diagnosis. J Clin Pathol 52:761–765

25. Mireskandari M, Kayser G, Hufnagal P, Schrader T, Kayser K (2004) Teleconsultation in diagnostic pathology: experience from Iran and Germany with the use of two European telepathology servers. J Telemed Telecare 10:307–308

26. Rashbass J, Furness P (2005) Telepathology: guidance from the Royal College of Pathologists. The Royal College of Pathologist, London. Available from http://www.rcpath.org/resources/pdf/G026-Telepathology-May05.pdf

27. Rosen PP (1989) Special report: perils problem and minimum requirements in shipping pathology slides. Am J Clin Pathol 91:348–354

28. Statistical Center of Iran (2007) National portal of statistic. Available from http://www.sci.org.ir/portal/faces/public/sci_en/sci_en.Glance/sci_en.health

29. Strauss JS, Felten CL, Okada DH, Marchevsky AM (1999) Virtual microscopy and public-key cryptography for Internet telepathology. J Telemed Telecare 5:105–110

30. Telemedicine in the Arab World (2000) Arab society of telemedicine. Available from http://www.itu.int/ITU-D/study_groups/SGP_1998-2002/SG2/Documents/2000/191E.doc
31. Weiss-Carrington P, Blount M, Kipreos B (1999) Telepathology between Richmond and Beckley Veterans Affairs Hospitals: report on the first 1000 cases. Telemed J 5:367–373
32. Wells CA, Sowter C (2000) Telepathology: a diagnostic tool for the millennium. J Pathol 191:1–7
33. Zem Technology (homepage on the Internet) (2008) Hoogblokland: Jordanian hospital acquires advanced Dutch Tele medicine system. August 07, 2008. Available from http://www.zem.com/tele-news.html

10

Telepathology in Japan

Takashi Sawai

A concept of telemedicine has been present from old days, and occasionally the necessity appeared in private and public lives. Recently, with the progression of information technology (IT), telemedicine has been of interest not only to the medical field but also to the government (Fig. 10.1). Telemedicine in Japan is comprised of mainly three factors: one is telehomecare, the second is teleradiology, and the third is telepathology, in which pathological and/or cytological images are transferred from medical institutes to the pathologists in remote institutes by cables (Fig. 10.2). Several causative factors that promote the telepathology in Japan are considered as shown in Fig. 10.3. One of the most important factors is a shortage of diagnostic pathologists. Before addressing telepathology itself, it is important to get a quick overview of diagnostic pathology in Japan. Then characteristic of Japanese telepathology is introduced and discussed from the medical, economical, and technological aspects for next development.

10.1
The Present Conditions of Japanese Diagnostic Pathology and the Background of Development of Telepathology

In 2004, there were 1,900 diagnostic pathologists recognized by the Japanese Society of Pathology (JSP), accounting for only 0.7% of the total number of physicians in Japan and showing only minimal growth (Fig. 10.4). This is the most severe doctor shortage of any field in Japan, followed in order by pediatricians, OB/GYNs, and anesthesiologists. As illustrated in Fig. 10.5, the ratio of pathologists to the general population is only about 20% of what it is in the United States. Pathologists have traditionally performed autopsies, biopsies, cytodiagnoses, and intraoperative rapid diagnosis. More recently, pathologists also run clinicopathological conferences (CPCs) for residents and clinicians. The most recent available JSP study shows that Japan's pathologists perform 32,000 autopsies, 5.5 million biopsies, 11 million cytodiagnoses, and 100,000 rapid diagnoses annually. All of these duties are increasing except autopsies year by year (Fig. 10.6), but the pathologists and their works has not been well

What is Telemedicine ?

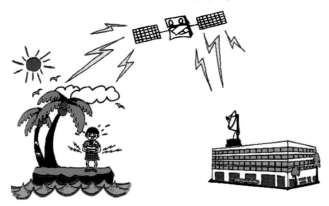

Fig. 10.1. What is telemedicine? The concept of telemedicine has been present in the social life from the old days

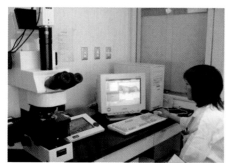

Sender (Physician Site)

Receiver (Pathologist Site)

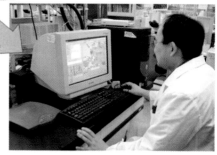

Transfer the Image

Fig. 10.2. Telepathology system via ISDN. This still image system is now the most spreading type and amounts to 75% of all systems in Japan. The pictures are transferred via ISDN. This system is introduced in 1992 between Tohoku University in Sendai city and Koritsu-Kesennuma Hospital in Kesennuma city in costal region, about 70 km distance

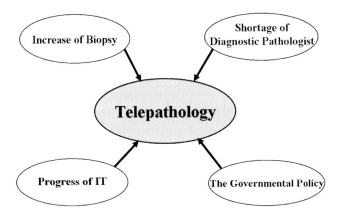

Fig. 10.3. Background of telepathology development. Among many factors that promote telepathology increase of biopsy samples, shortage of diagnostic pathologists, IT progress, and policy by the Governmental are major factors

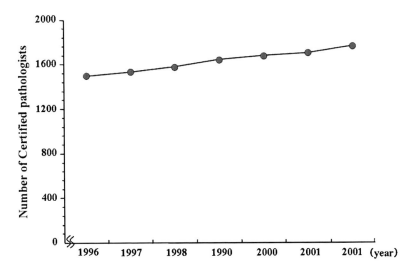

Fig. 10.4. Number of diagnostic pathologists. The number of pathologists increases gradually but still insufficient in Japan

recognized in Japanese society in spite of their important roles (Fig. 10.7). For example, the situation in northern part of Japan (Tohoku Area) is illustrated in Fig. 10.8. Despite having 868 hospitals with 200 or more beds, full-time pathologists are almost exclusively confined to university hospitals and major hospitals in the prefectural capitals. Even large hospitals in other major cities rarely have full-time pathologists on staff [12–14].

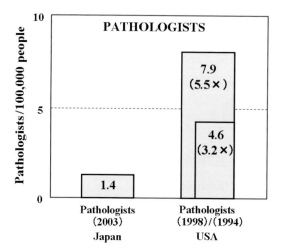

Fig. 10.5. Comparison of pathologist' number between Japan and USA. The numerical ratio of pathologists to the general population is only about 20% compared with one in the USA

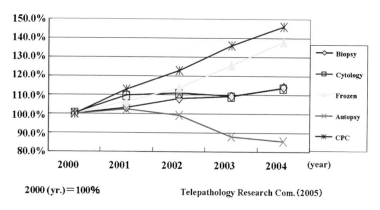

Fig. 10.6. Number of pathological duties in Japan. Pathologist's duties are comprised of biopsy, cytology, frozen rapid diagnosis, autopsy, and clinical pathological conference. The number of duties increases year by year except for autopsy

For this reason, biopsies and cytodiagnoses are often outsourced to university, public, or private laboratories. Generally it takes about several days to a week to get a diagnosis. Under these circumstances, it is impossible to perform intra-operative rapid diagnosis for decision of a next surgical step, especially on a cutoff margin, and has been left to the experience and intuition of the surgeons, as shown in Fig. 10.9. A veteran surgeon's judgment can be accurate relatively, but, in case of new and inexperienced cases or tumors with unclear boundaries, even experienced surgeons hesitate to carry out the operation. Tumors not fully

Have you ever heard the name of pathologist ?

Do you know the duty of pathologist ?

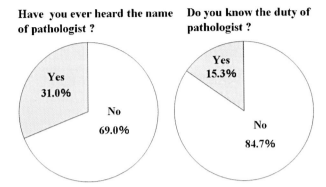

Yes 31.0%

No 69.0%

Yes 15.3%

No 84.7%

Fig. 10.7. Public consciousness relating pathologist and their duties in Japan. Pathologists and their duties are surprisingly not known publicly in Japan

Tohoku Area (Japanese Northern Part)

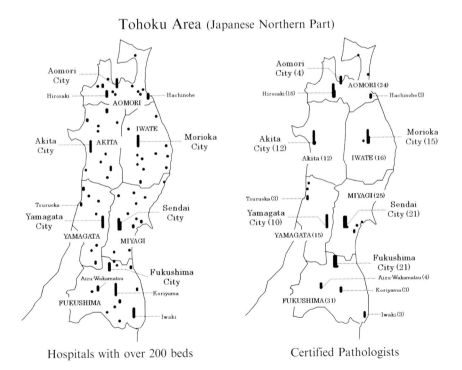

Hospitals with over 200 beds

Certified Pathologists

Fig. 10.8. Distribution of hospitals with more than 200 beds (*left*) and hospitals with certified pathologists (*right*). The number of pathologists is very small in northern part of Japan and most of all converge into university and large hospitals in large cities

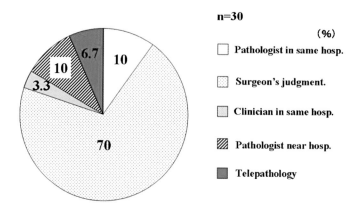

Fig. 10.9. In case of necessity who diagnoses rapidly? In the hospital without pathologists, quick decision related to next step in operation is dependent on surgeon's experience and intuition

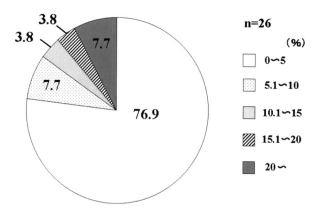

Fig. 10.10. The ratio of intraoperative rapid diagnosis. Ratio of cases requiring intraoperative diagnosis to all operations is 5% (surgeons' comment)

excised will surely recur. From a survey of surgeons with 15 or more years of experience, it was revealed that 3–10% of past cases (5% on average) require the intraoperative rapid diagnosis (Fig. 10.10).

10.2
The History of IT and Telepathology in Japan

The background of telepathology development in Japan is shown in Fig. 10.3. Among them, most noticeable and influential fields in development of information technologies are the spread of the Internet. Microscopic imaging, for example, has seen enormous advances with the digitization of images, and it has become possible to quickly and easily transfer images to distant locations. However, pathologists who diagnose by optical microscopy systems have felt a great deal of resistance to image-only diagnosis, more than troublesome, and not sufficiently developed systems. Indeed, early telepathology images were vastly inferior to microscopic images and had a risk of misdiagnoses. An additional problem was that it took a longer time to diagnose with still images compared with optical microscopy, and the frustration occurred to both clinicians and diagnosticians. For these reasons, many pathologists were not enthusiastic about the practicality of telepathology.

In 1982, what was probably the world's first telepathology in color experiment was carried out by Dr. Hiroshi Sakaguchi of Keio University in Tokyo [7]. This test linked the university to a hospital in Hachioji (also in Tokyo). A quarter century after this experiment using analog phone lines, fiber optics and digital images are becoming the norm. Almost a decade later, at the 23rd Japan Medical Congress in 1991, the Kyoto Prefectural University of Medicine linked with Yosanoumi Hospital (on the Japan Sea side) to demonstrate telepathology, which was subsequently added to the university's normal operations. The National Cancer Center also hooked up its main hospital in Tsukiji, Tokyo, with Hospital East in Kashiwa, Chiba, and Yamagata University connected its Faculty of Medicine with the University Hospital via optical fiber. The following year, at the 81st meeting of the JSP, Tohoku University was linked with Sendai City Hospital through optical fibers for a video (motion picture) telepathology experiment [11]. At this stage, each facility was researching and developing its own telepathology formats.

10.3
Recent Governmental Policy and Activity to Telepathology

Recently, the prevalence of telepathology has been accelerating. Among the changing societal factors for the development of telepathology are continuing the condition of shortage of diagnostic pathologists (Fig. 10.4), the prevalence of the Internet, and the societal shift to computerization in social activity, including medical filed, medical accidents, and patients' increasing desire for a second opinion. In addition, the establishment of a Telemedicine Research Committee by the Health and Welfare Ministry (the current Ministry of Health, Labor, and Welfare, or MLHW) cannot be ignored. The research group, initially headed by Dr. Shigekoto Kaihara of the University of Tokyo (currently dean of the graduate school of the International University of Health and Welfare), researched homecare, teleradiology, and telepathology. Another significant event in the history of telepathology came in 2000, when telepathology was

included as an insured health-care service. This was followed by the expansion
of diagnostic facilities in 2003. The MLHW's official acceptance of telepathology
represented a change from its previous policy of recognizing only direct, face-
to-face medicine, and this was a major impetus for the spread of telepathology. The telepathology research committee supported by MLHW defined that
telepathology is to do something related to a medical action associated with
medical practice, education, and research from the distant area on the basis of
information of macro- and microscopical images.

Although some aspects of telepathology such as added fees required for
equipment and telecommunication are still unclear, recent surveys have shown
that the usage of telepathology is steadily, although gradually, increasing. In
2004, 55 facilities were linked with 120 hospitals and clinics to provide telepathological services for nearly 2,600 cases (Fig. 10.11). Apart from the telemedicine
research group supported by the government, pathologists, physicians, cytologists, vendor, and developer of private company established the group named
the "Japanese Research Society of Telepathology and Telepathology Informatics"
(JRST-TI) in 2000, had made a guideline for Japanese usage in 2003 [19], and
changed the name to the "Japanese Research Society of Telepathology Virtual
Microscopy" (JRST ċ VM), now examining a guideline for a telecytology and
application for virtual microscopy.

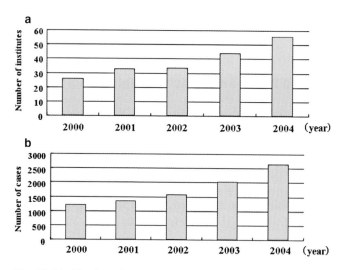

Fig. 10.11. Number of institutes practicing telepathology and the number of cases. Institutes
and number of cases practicing telepathology increase gradually year by year

10.4
The Purpose of Japanese Telepathology, Especially Intraoperative Rapid Diagnosis

In Europe and the United States, telepathology is used widely in consultations, but in Japan, it is overwhelmingly used for intraoperative rapid diagnosis (Fig. 10.12). One of the reasons for this difference is that telepathology in Japan began from rapid diagnosis under the auspices of the MLHW. This intensive government support for telepathology is characteristic and may be different from other countries in the world. The other reason for development is the latent clinical desire for rapid diagnosis for telepathology. In the future, because of patients' increased consciousness in medicine and a spate of recent medical lawsuits, it seems likely that telepathology will be used increasingly in consultations and second opinions and other purposes relating images.

Generally, rapid telepathological diagnosis is used for diagnosis of malignant tumors and metastasis, and for confirmation of cutoff margin whether tumor is still left or not (Fig. 10.13) [23]. I, here, introduce two surgical cases, one is a need for a further resection and the other is finished without additional excision in a short time owing to diagnosis of telepathology (Figs. 10.14 and 10.15). These are the large benefits of telepathology viewing from the point of medical and economical aspects.

In the past, the MLHW requested a study of the relationship between rapid diagnosis and the recurrence of tumors. In other words, the ministry wanted to know with what frequency cancers recurred, as rapid diagnosis had not been performed. When it became clear that there was no hope of cooperation from

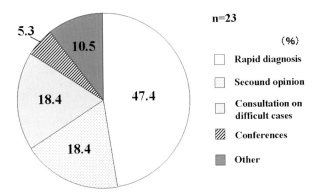

Fig. 10.12. The purpose of telepathology. The telepathology is used for intraoperative rapid diagnosis, second opinion, consultation, and pathological and clinical pathological conference

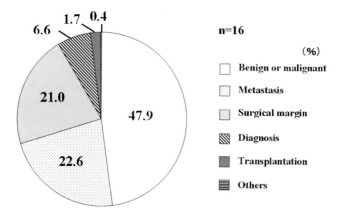

Fig. 10.13. The purpose of intraoperative rapid diagnosis. Diagnosis whether the tumor is malignant or benign, confirmation of metastasis, and cutoff margin are major purposes of intraoperative rapid diagnosis for decision of next step quickly

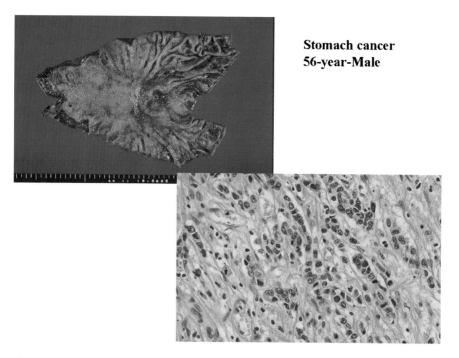

Stomach cancer 56-year-Male

Fig. 10.14. Intraoperative rapid diagnosis performed in telepathology. The patient was a 56-year-old male. He underwent the operation for stomach cancer. Intraoperative rapid diagnosis in telepathology revealed the cancer residue in cutoff margin at esophago–cardiac junction, and further excision was performed

Transferred Image   Permanent Image

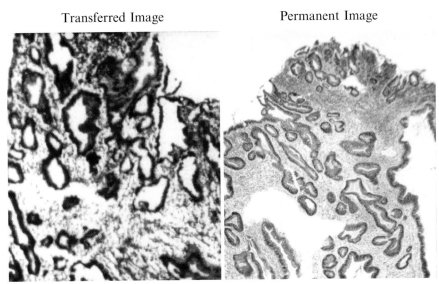

66-year-Female
Clin. Diag.: Carcinoma of common bile duct
Pathol. Diag.: Adenoma, not malignant

Fig. 10.15. Intraoperative rapid diagnosis by telepathology. The patient was a 66-year-old female. She underwent the operation for carcinoma of common bile duct. Intraoperative quick diagnosis by telepathology showed that the tumor was adenoma, not malignancy, against preoperative clinical diagnosis. Operation was finished without further wide resection. She is well now

medical practitioners, the ministry asked, instead, for a report of the percentage of surgeons' requests for rapid diagnosis. Improperly or incompletely removed tumors always recur, endangering patient's lives. But that is not all. Recurrence obviously places enormous physical and emotional burdens on patients and their families and also wastes valuable medical time and resources. Studies have shown that initial operations on gastrointestinal cancers like stomach and colon cancer cost about $18,000 (Table 10.1) and that subsequent therapies in the case of recurrence are never less expensive. On the contrary, Tanita (Japanese respiratory surgeon) reports that using video-assisted thoracoscopic surgery (VATS) for a rapid lung cancer diagnosis and followed by the excision of the same pathological lesion, if necessary, lead to a saving of $4500 compared with performing two separate surgeries [16]. From these facts, it is clear that the pathological intraoperative rapid diagnosis not only improves in patients' prognosis but also brings an economical saving as intensively desired by the MLHW.

Table 10.1. Payment for hospitalization of carcinoma operation and the recurrence

Age (year) (Sex)	Disease (result)	Operating mood	Hospital stay (months)	Hospital fee ($)
67 (male)	Colon cancer	Colectomy	2	11,300
	Recurrence (dead: after 3 years)	Ope (–)	3	18,253
86 (male)	Stomach cancer	Total gas-torectomy	1	19,600
	Recurrence (dead: after 1 year)	Ope (–)	2	9282
63 (male)	Stomach cancer	Total gas-torectomy	2	23,905
	Recurrence (dead: after 2 years)	Ope (–)	1	10,124

Charge to be paid is not so different between the first operation and the recurrence, that is to say, the recurrence of tumor brings a large economical burden as well as time, labor, and patient's life

10.5
Development of Infrastructure and Telepathology Systems in Japan

Telepathology systems require both hardware and software. Hardware is mainly IT dependent, including communications infrastructure, digital cameras, computers, and microscopes. Software applications provide the tools to effectively use this infrastructure. In its infancy, telepathology relied entirely on analog phone lines. Integrated Services Digital Network (ISDN) subsequently became available, then multiple ISDN lines were bundled together, and most recently the field has begun to move to asymmetric digital subscriber lines (ADSL) and optical fiber cable. These developments have vastly increased the amount of transferable data (Fig. 10.16). Mobile telepathology is also being developed. Although it initially relied on communications satellites, mobile telepathology benefits from the technological advances seen, for example, in mobile phones, which are now able to receive image data on the move. However, issues including image quality, operability, and internationalization remain unresolved.

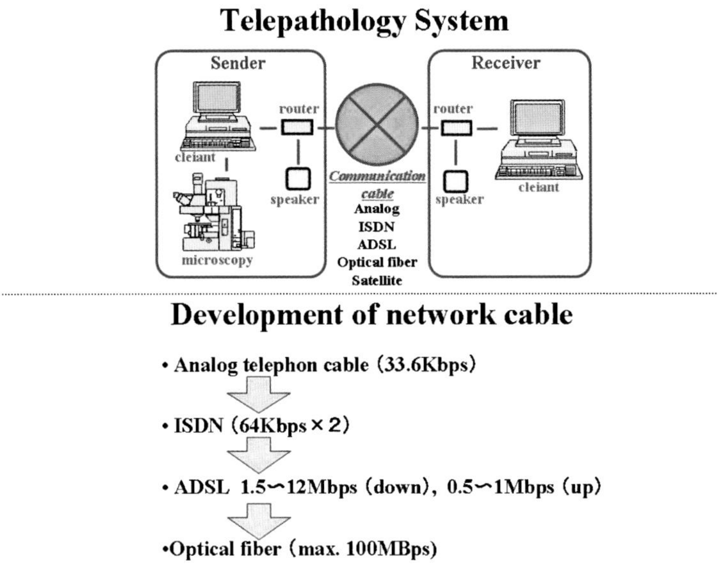

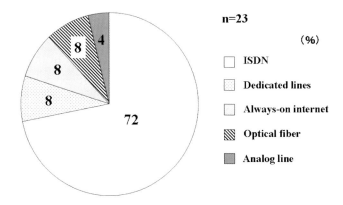

Fig. 10.16. Telepathology system (*upper*) and network development (*lower*). In short time, network cable has developed from analog cable through ISDN, ADSL, to recent optical fiber

Fig. 10.17. The infrastructural cables used for telepathology (2002). Although the ISDN was most utilized cable for telepathology in 2002, the broadband (ADSL and optical fiber) may take place now, including still, video, and virtual pictures in a short time

As shown in Fig. 10.17, rather old data, the overwhelming majority of telepathology systems rely on the transfer of still images over ISDN lines. Although in most cases the pathologists on diagnostic site is able to select the field by remote control, some systems still require the physician who requests the diagnosis on sending site to operate system by himself. Analog telepathology formats using

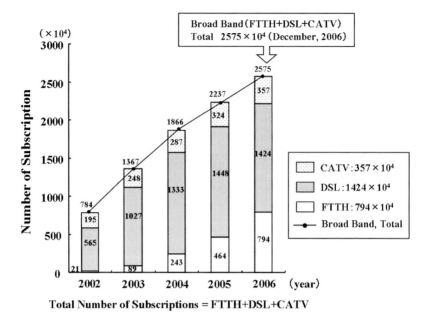

Fig. 10.18. Number of broadband subscriptions. Number of subscriptions of broadband including CATV, DSL, and FTTH increases rapidly in Japan by the aid of the Japanese government

telephone lines still exist, but they are disappearing rapidly in Japan. In their places, formats using broadband Internet connections (ADSL and optical fiber) have appeared, and, in the context of Japan's e-Japan Strategy and u-Japan Policy, expectations are high for their future progress. At the end of 2006, about 26 million families subscribed for broadband usage (Fig. 10.18). In particular, video telepathology via optical fiber allows the diagnostician to select the viewing fields freely and operate the equipment by themselves, meaning that the observation process is nearly identical to checking specimens under a conventional microscope directly (Fig. 10.19). This video telepathology has brought astonishing effect on saving time for intraoperative rapid diagnosis, as shown in Table 10.2 [15].

10.6
Telepathology Applications in Medical Field

As noted earlier, telepathology is currently being used in intraoperative rapid diagnosis, provision of second opinions, consultations, and conferences (Fig. 10.12). Rapid diagnosis employs telepathology to diagnose whether malignancy or not,

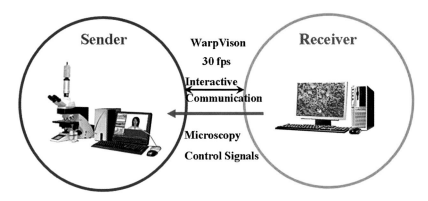

Fig. 10.19. Video telepathology system. Selecting the visual field and focusing are operated by observer freely, as well as direct optical microscopy using remote controller via optical fiber

Table 10.2. Intraoperative rapid diagnosis by video image via optical fiber

	Telepathology via video system (11.1.2004 to 1.15.2005)			
No.	Organ	Sample Size (mm)	Time (min)	Diagnosis
1	Margin, pancreas	20 × 15	3	No carcinoma infiltration
2	Margin, stomach	8 × 20	3	No carcinoma infiltration
3	Margin, stomach	5 × 35	6	No carcinoma infiltration
4	Margin, stomach	10 × 7	6	No carcinoma infiltration
5	Margin, stomach	12 × 8	4	No carcinoma infiltration
6	Margin, duodenum margin, esophagus	3 × 85 × 9	43	No carcinoma infiltration
7	Margin, stomach	5 × 10	7	No carcinoma infiltration
8	Margin, pancreas	20 × 15	3	No carcinoma infiltration

Mean time—4.3 min/slide

The pathologist can freely select the visual field as well as adjusting the focus of the slides glass on the table of optical microscopy from the remote institute as if seeing the optical microscopy directly. Mean time of intraoperative rapid diagnosis by video image is accomplished in 4.4 min/case, very short compared with still image in 35 min/case

classify tumors, confirm metastasis, and decide the surgical margin. Second opinions are required for the reconfirmation of borderline diagnostic tumors and for therapeutic selection from various ones. Furthermore, it appears that rather than extremely difficult cases, telepathology is used more frequently to determine whether a gastric tissue biopsy is group III or IV – in other words, whether or not an immediate operation is necessary. Telepathology is also becoming increasingly popular for breast cancer diagnosis [3,8] and second opinions from the point of cosmetic therapy as well as medical one.

Several facilities have CPCs by teleconferencing system, for example, Tokyo Medical University's internal CPC between medical school in Shinjyuku and Hachoji Hospital, and Iwate Medical University's conferences for interns with the Kuji Prefectural Hospital in the Sanriku area (on sea side) over a steep mountain, using the teleconferencing technologies. We had a teleconference linking 301 hospitals in Beijing in China over the Internet (Fig. 10.20) [22] and also had a video teleconference with Ryukyus University in Okinawa, the most southern

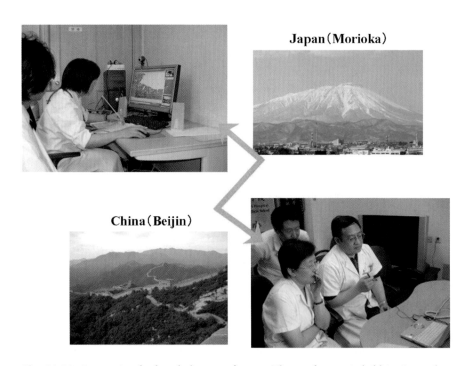

Fig. 10.20. International telepathology conference. The conference is held in September 2006 between Japan (Morioka) and China (Beijing), via cables of optical fiber at Japan site and ADSL at China site

islands area in Japan, about 2,000 km away from our IWATE Medical University, via optical fiber.

Telepathology is applied for community medicine and for the treatments in many fields. One of them is for operation of pulmonary cancer [1], associated with smoking, which is increasing in number (women in particular). Another is transplant medicine [4,5], for which there are not enough specialists in Japan. Second opinions are often sought regarding surgical procedure in hemopathies requiring emergency treatment, and breast cancer or prostatic cancer. Recently, the telecytology has also been paid attention via Internet or optical fiber [24,25]. For now, suffice it to say that telepathology is effective in many situations and offers outstanding medical and economic benefits.

10.7
The Telepathology System in Future

10.7.1
The Government Strategy to Telepathology

As it is impossible to increase the number of pathologists rapidly in the near future in Japan, telepathology for elevation of a medical level is necessary. Japan's e-Japan Strategy and u-Japan Policy assure that the nation's optical fiber infrastructure will continue to grow. Given this, discussions on the future of telepathology can be predicated on the existence of increasingly universal broadband telecommunications. It seems likely that, depending on the cable infrastructure of optical fiber, telepathology using video (motion) and/or many still images may well become the norm. On the while, virtual microscopy, in another word, the digital microscopy, has been increasingly introduced recently in Japan, because the MLHW endeavor to promote "the cancer control strategy" in which digital microscopy is recommended for establishing the consultation system via web servers (Fig. 10.21). MLHW established the new group for standardizing the medical levels, including diagnoses and therapeutics. By the governmental quick action, about 100 medical institutes introduced the digital microscopy in only half a year. Probably the number of digital microscopes in Japan is second next to USA in the world. This digital microscope is also available for the education such as histological and pathological studies and already used in several medical schools, which has brought the discussion, in medical education, whether traditional optical microscopy is necessary or not in the practical training for medical students [2,17,18]. However, the digital microscope now requires a long time to load the images for using intraoperative rapid diagnosis.

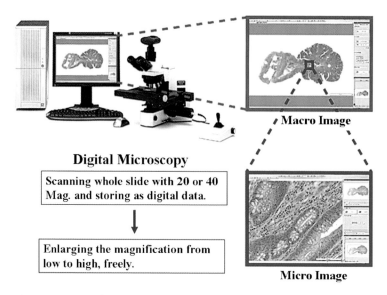

Fig. 10.21. Digital microscopy system. The system of digital microscopy, called scan micros-copy, is now broadly introduced in Japan for diagnostic consultation and education, especially in the field of "cancer control strategy," promoted by the Japanese government

Mobile technology has made wireless pathological diagnosis possible and eventually should be able to transfer images between the Japanese mainland and outlying islands, as well as internationally. But for a small volume of transfer-able capacity, mobile telepathology is not practical but still in the experimental stage [21]. Internet-based telepathology serves as a stopgap in areas where opti-cal fiber is still not available, but the use of the Internet raises security concerns. Internet-based telepathology includes both the use of e-mail file attachments and the server-based file transfer [6].

Three kinds of telepathology systems are considerable in Japan: first, most popular system is using e-mail with attachment of the figures for international communication as well as for domestic area without broadband cables; the sec-ond is video (motion) images telepathology system by broadband cables such as ADSL and optical fiber; and the last is digital microscope, using uploaded images in web server for consultation and/or second opinion, and also for the medical education. When broadband Internet becomes ubiquitous, it would be ideal for video and uploaded images to be toggled with a single click so that both could be used in rapid diagnosis or consultations for necessity (Fig. 10.22).

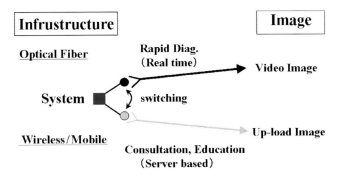

Fig. 10.22. Combination system of video and digital images. The combination telepathology system is applicable for both intraoperative rapid diagnosis and consultation and/or education

10.7.2
Technological Development of DVDs and the Imaging Compression Technology

As broadband image transfer becomes possible, the development of equipment to send and save massive amounts of data becomes necessary. As the number of pixels in digital images increases, their precision improves. However, these higher-quality images also require greater storage space; especially virtual slides, a recent development in pathological imaging, are particularly large. Even if a few slides could be saved on, as the number of cases increases, much higher capacity storage also becomes necessary. Recent technologies allow these images to be compressed, saved, and decompressed again later for use. Hopefully, these compression technologies will continue to develop and evolve day by day.

10.8
Problems Relating the Prevalence of Telepathology in Japan

Telepathology in Japan began as an expedient way to use IT to compensate for the shortage of diagnostic pathologists. In this sense, the progress of telepathology has been quite spectacular as Japan's IT strategy. It appears that if only the number of diagnostic pathologists would increase, telepathology's original goal could be reached. However, it is highly unlikely that such an increase will happen anytime soon. Furthermore, telepathology reveals the superior effect more than we expected in early stage, by which excellent images are useful not only for diagnosis but also for image storage as digital memory in computer without color fade, saving spaces of slide glass and also using the images at any

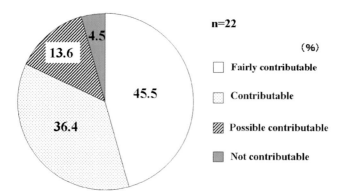

Fig. 10.23. Evaluation of telepathology for community medicine by doctors. More than 95% of surgeons consider that the telepathology is contributable on community medicine

time easily without wasting time, transferring by cable, or transporting by USB flash memories.

For the forefront of medicine, frequent occurrence of medical lawsuits, electronic medical records promoted by national policies, and the image-based e-learning [9] and/or researches [20], telepathology is poised for continued growth and development, with the improvement of the related infrastructure and hardware. Figure 10.23 represents the surgeon's comments related to the role of telepathology on community medicine [10]. More than 95% surgeons consider that telepathology is contributable or community medicine and want to use it, if economical problem is settled.

To contribute the best to the medical field, it is imperative that the governmental, academic, and industrial sectors work together to form a shared future vision.

10.9
Summary

- Telemedicine, developed based on the progress of IT, mainly comprises telehomecare, teleradiology, and telepathology.
- Telepathology in Japan begun in 1990s and developed because of shortage of pathologist, remarkable development of information technology, and relaxation of law, and by the governmental policy on IT. Now the number of institutes practicing telepathology amounts to 55 and cases are 2,600 in 1 year.
- The purposes of telepathology are intraoperative rapid diagnosis, consultation and/or second opinion, clinical pathological conference, etc.; the most urgent requirement being intraoperative rapid diagnosis, which is useful for

confirmation of cancer, metastasis, and decision of cutoff margin to decide following operative steps immediately.

- Japanese telepathology style for intraoperative diagnosis is probably rare and characteristic in the world but brought the large economical as well as medical effects.

- Infrastructure of Japanese telepathology begun in early stage via analog cable and, through ISDN and ADSL, reached the optical fiber. Telepathology systems also have changed their styles from still images to motion (video) and/ or virtual ones, which are wanted for rapid diagnosis in operation by surgeons. Virtual microscopy is required for consultation and education.

References

1. Eguchi K, Kobayshi K (2008) 4-1 Survey on the application of telepathology to pulmonary cancer. In Sawai T (ed) Telepathology in Japan – development and practice. Celc, Morioka. pp.117–122
2. Furuya K, Maeda T, Nakasato K (2005) Virtual slide and its wide applications including pathology diagnosis (in Japanese). Jpn J Cancer Clin 51:727–731
3. Hufnagl P, Bayer G, Oberbamscheidt P, et al (2001) Comparison of different telepathology solutions for primary frozen section diagnostic. Anal Cell Pathol 21:161–167
4. Ito H, Adachi H, Taniyama K, et al (1994) Telepathology is available for transplantation–pathology in Japan using integrated, low-cost, and high quality system. Mod Pathol 7: 801–805
5. Ito H, Shomori K, Adachi H, Arihiro K, Sasaki N, Taniyama K (2005) Application of telepathology for clinical organ-transplantation (in Japanese). Jpn J Cancer Clin 51:669–674
6. Iyama K, Honda Y, Ikeda K, et al (2005) A useful consultation software for "P to P" telepathology (in Japanese). Jpn J Cancer Clin 51:691–698
7. Kawakita I, Senda R, Sakaguchi H (1983) Experiment study of Hitachi telepathology system (in Japanese). J Med Technol 27:1557–1559
8. Moriya T, Endoh M, Watanabe M, Sawai T (2005) Telepathology for breast lesions (in Japanese). Jpn J Cancer Clin 51:675–678
9. Ohshiro M, Tsuchihashi Y, Shiraishi T (2005) Consultation using a center system – expression of telepathology use such as diagnosis and education (in Japanese). Jpn J Cancer Clin 51:705–710
10. Saito K, Takahashi T, Chiba G, Sawai T (2005) Development of medical information sharing web system for telepathology and tele-consultation (in Japanese). Jpn J Cancer Clin 51:711–719
11. Sawai T (1994) Experimental report of telepathology by HDTV via optical fiber (in Japanese). In: Kyogku M, Nagura H (eds) Research society of telepathology in Sendai. New Media, Tokyo, pp. 39–102
12. Sawai T (2005) Telepathology in Japan (in Japanese). Jpn J Cancer Clin 51:649–656
13. Sawai T (2008) 1-1 The state of telepathology in Japan. In Sawai T (ed) Telepathology in Japan – development and practice. Celc, Morioka. pp. 3–9
14. Sawai T, Goto K, Watanabe M, Endoh W, Ogata K, Nagura H (1999) Constructing a local district telepathology network in Japan. Diagnosis of intraoperative frozen sections via

telepathology over an integrated service digital network and the national television standard committee system. Anal Quant Cytol Histol 21:81–84

15. Sawai T, Noda Y, Kumagai K, Matsumura I (2005) Pilot study of telepathology in dynamic image by public optical fiber (in Japanese). Jpn J Cancer Clin 51:699–703

16. Tanita T, Kobayashi K, Hasegawa T (2005) The medical and financial effectiveness of telepathology systems for an intraoperative quick diagnosis for surgery for lung cancer. Jpn J Cancer Clin 51:663–667

17. Tofukuji I, Sawai T (2004) A development plan of the next generation telepathology system. Telemed e-Health J 10:S115

18. Tofukuji I, Sawai T, Tsuchihashi Y (2006) Recent development of telepathology in Japan. Proceeding of 8th European Congress on Telepathology and 2nd International Congress on Virtual Microscopy

19. Tsuchihashi Y, Sawai T (2005) Establishing guidelines for practical telepathology in Japan (in Japanese). Jpn J Cancer Clin 51:721–725

20. Uzuki M (2008) 5-3 Research application for telepathology. In Sawai T (ed) Telepathology in Japan – development and practice. Celc, Morioka. pp. 117–122

21. Uzuki M, Sawai T (2006) Experimental study of virtual telepathology system under mobile environment for ubiquitous telepathology (in Japanese). Igaku No Ayumi (J Clin Res Med) 218:247–250

22. Uzuki M, Sawai T (2007) Internationalization of telepathology-Internet pathology conference between Japan and China (in Japanese). Igaku No Ayumi (J Clin Res Med) 220:848–852

23. Watanabe M, Endoh M, Moriya T, Sawai T (2005) Experience of more than 1,000 telepathology cases in Tohoku University Hospital (in Japanese). Jpn J Cancer Clin 51:679–686

24. Yamashiro K, Kawamura N, Matsubayashi S, et al (2004) Telecytology in Hokkaido Island, Japan: results of primary telecytodiagnosis of routine cases. Cytopathology 15:221–227

25. Yamashiro K, Suzuki H, Taira K, et al (2005) Practical use of telecytology-contribution to community medicine (in Japanese). Jpn J Cancer Clin 51:687–690

Telepathology in Hungary

M. Cserneky, B. Szende, L. Fónyad, and T. Krenács

"The greatest threat to information is not using it"
—e-consulting, Symantec

11.1
Historical Background

A special structure of health care and hospital system was established after World War II in Hungary, corresponding to that of the Soviet Union. Altogether 80 hospitals, including university, county, and municipal hospitals as well as National Institutes (of Oncology, Rheumatology, Psychiatry, Neurosurgery, Pulmonology, Cardiology, Dermatology, and Venerology), were part of this system. All of these hospitals and institutes run at least 400 hospital beds, and according to the law a histopathology department had to be operated in each of them. This concept generated a highly fragmented, irrational, and expensive structure in a small central European country of 93,000 km^2 (Fig. 11.1). Pathology service was already understaffed, which became even more emphasized by the regionally uneven dispersal of professionals. Number of registered pathologists was and still is about 200, with more than 30% of them working at six university departments and in departments of the national institutes. Pathology departments of county hospitals are still run by two to three pathologists, and most of the municipal hospitals depend on a "one-man" pathology service.

By the late 1980s, the system of pathology service got close to collapsing. The number of pathologists remained virtually unchanged, but the average age of them increased steadily because of the lack of young residents and the emigration of middle-aged specialists to Western Europe. Increasing numbers of pathologies became "one-man" departments, and more and more small hospitals were left without a pathologist. Liberalization of some functions of the health-care system in Hungary after the political changes in 1990 did not result in the expected benefits to the structure of the pathology service.

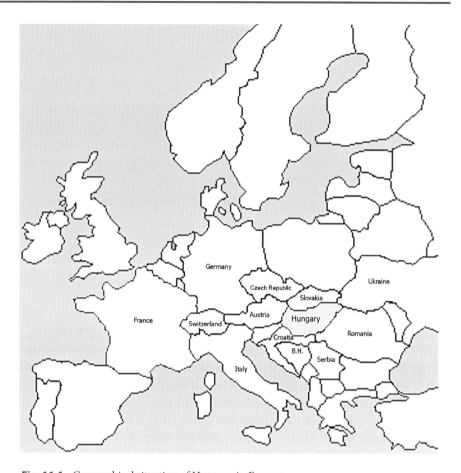

Fig. 11.1. Geographical situation of Hungary in Europe

Despite the gradually increasing number of tasks in modern pathology, the number of pathologists and pathology departments remained unchanged, which conserved the obstacles in consultations and limited the chances of pathologists in one- or two-men departments to participate in postgraduate courses. Shortage of financial resources just aggravated the situation. Leading Hungarian pathologists sought for solutions to maintain the level of practicing pathology and keep pace with international standards. Since the principles of telepathology were known to several Hungarian pathologists, one of the possibilities was to try exploiting its potential benefits under the special circumstances of Hungarian medical care [12,15].

The main goals for introducing telepathology in practice in Hungary were the following:

- To make available fast and high-quality histopathological diagnosis for surgical departments in hospitals lacking pathologists
- To reduce duration of hospitalization by avoiding delays in consultation as a result of mailing histological sections or blocks
- To avoid unnecessary extension of anesthesia in case of intraoperative frozen sections
- To ensure quality control by direct consultation and facilitate permanent postgraduate teaching supported by an established database of histopathological cases, including pathomorphological image collections

11.2
First Steps to Introduce Telepathology in Hungary

The first attempt to start telepathology in Hungary was made in 1994 by the Department of Pathology of the MI Central Hospital, Budapest, as peripheral diagnostic unit (project leader: Dr Peter Gombás) and the first Department of Pathology and Experimental Cancer Research, Semmelweis University, Budapest, as consultant center (project leader: Dr Béla Szende). The diagnostic unit was equipped with an Olympus consulting microscope and a video camera of 450 lines horizontal resolution. The consulting center had an IBM PC486 with 8 MB RAM operative memory using a software, developed by the firm ADDA, running a Windows system. Images produced by this card were 8-bit BMP files with a 256 color depth and 640 × 480 pixels resolution and 300 kB size, stored on a file server. The sender site was equipped with an IBM PC486. In the first phase of the system, a commercial modem and its software with 9.6 kbaud transmission speed were applied through analog telephone line to connect the two work stations. This system resulted in file transmitting of single static images chosen by the sender. Transmission time was rather long, and therefore the consultation was of limited value.

As a further step, supported by the Foundation for Leukaemic Children in Hungary, a 2B + D structured ISDN phone line with 128 kbps information transmitting capacity was used, securing digital access. Using a Windows-based software, with a Bitfield video communication system (BVCS) H.320 coding standard and FCIF standard 325 × 288 pixel resolution digitalizing card, the transfer of live, properly assessable video images amended with verbal telephone communication resulted in a relatively fast and successful consultation of histological, immunohistochemical, and cytological samples [9,10]. The establishment of the above system was partly supported by the Hungarian National Committee for Technology Development. However, the extension of the network and further improvements in instrumentation needed financial and advisory support from the European Union.

11.3
Further Developments Supported by the European Union

Based on the available instrumentation, infrastructure, and skilled personnel, a group of pathologists and surgeons in Budapest applied for grant support of the FP-4 Research Program of the European Union, which included the Interactive Histopathology Consultation Network (Interpath—PL-96112). The application was managed by Varimed Ltd. (head: Dr Sándor Vári) and led to success in 1998. The supervisor of this and the following projects on behalf of the European Union was Professor Gerard Brugal (Grenoble, France). This project supported the establishment of two up-to-date and complete telepathology sender and receiver stations, one at the first Department of Pathology and Experimental Cancer Research and one at the Department of Transplantation and Surgery, Semmelweis University in Budapest. The equipment consisted of Axioplan 2 microscopes (Zeiss, Jena, Germany), Sony DXC-390 P cameras, Matrox Intellicam Cards, and Samba TPS 7.05 software (Samba Technologies, France). The same ISDN phone line was used as described earlier. Built-in microphones and macrocameras secured the verbal and video communication without extra telephone connection.

The aim of Interpath (between 1998 and 2000) was to test the new system enabling these two departments to assess intraoperative frozen sections, which were made at the surgical department and diagnosed at the distant department of pathology. This highly successful project allowed proceeding with the second step, that is, to join the Regional and International Integrated Telemedicine Network for Medical Assistance in end-stage diseases and organ transplantation (Retransplant—HC-IN4028, from 2000 till 2002). Retransplant extended the telepathology network to three more departments of pathology in the country and also supported the diagnostic work of radiology departments by allowing teleradiology. Encouraged by the success of this program, a nationwide teleconsultation system could be established within the BePrO (best practice in pathology and oncology) project (between 2001 and 2002) of the European Union. BePrO was cosponsored and integrated in Hungary by the Hungarian Division of IAP (president: Prof. Dr. Anna Kádár).

11.4
Structure and Function of Bepro in Hungary

11.4.1
General Considerations

About 600,000–700,000 histopathological diagnoses are made in Hungary annually, and in 5–10% of the cases a second opinion is requested. Geographical distribution of hospitals in the country and the decreasing number of skilled pathologists urged the construction of a telepathology network covering the whole country. Priority was given to six county hospitals (Budapest, Eger, Kecskemét, Kistarcsa, Székesfehérvár, and Szombathely) and university departments (first and second Departments of Pathology, Semmelweis University; Department of Pathology, University of Szeged), as well as to small municipal hospitals, which needed continuous diagnostic support from county hospitals and university departments (Fig. 11.2). Furthermore, telepathology consultations between Hungarian pathologists and European experts were also desirable, particularly in difficult diagnostic cases of tumors demanding critical prognostic and therapeutic considerations.

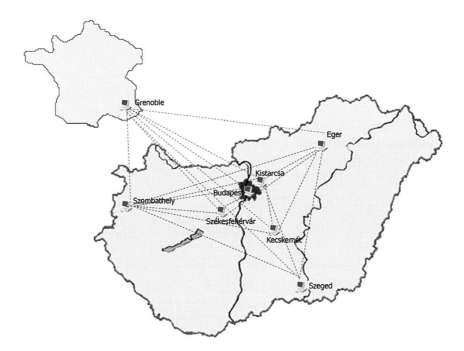

Fig. 11.2. Telepathology network in Hungary (BePro), connected with Grenoble, France

11.4.2
Structure of the Telepathology Stations

Three university departments and six county hospital departments of pathology were included in the project. Bilateral consultations were performed between the various stations, utilizing the possibilities provided by both ISDN telephone lines and Internet. All clinical data of the patients were stored and sent in using an eForm (HTML/XML). The images, sent to the consultant pathologist, were put in DICOM (digital imaging and communications in medicine) form and stored on a server operated by the European Coordinator's Institute in Grenoble (France) and also on the consultants' stations, strictly keeping to the regulations of data protection. Still images digitalized with a Sony DCX390P camera at a resolution of 700 × 600 DPI were attached to the eForms, which became part of the consulting department's protocols. All participants and the organizing department (first Department of Pathology and Experimental Cancer Research, Semmelweis University, Budapest) registered the consultations in order to document and evaluate their performance in support of the pathologists' diagnostic service.

11.4.3
Function of the Bepro Project Between November 2001 and June 2002

During the above period, online consultation was performed in 161 diagnostic cases, needing second opinion by transmitting of 786 images. Average consultation time was 13.18 min (Table 11.1). Pathological diagnoses mainly on tumors were consulted in the following organs and tissues: brain, intestines, skin, bone, bone marrow, breast, stomach, peripheral nerve, soft tissue, liver, uterus, parathyroid glands, thyroid gland, adrenal gland, mesentery, salivary glands, lymph nodes, ovary, pancreas, retroperitoneal tissues, lung, kidney, and organs of the oral cavity (Fig. 11.3). The most frequently consulted tumors were those of the skin, breast, and thyroid gland. Figure 11.4 shows examples for transmitted and stored histological images. Discrepancies between the diagnoses of the sender and the consultant department were found in altogether 14 cases, including tumors of the lung, breast, skin, and soft tissues, as shown in Fig. 11.5. A database was created from the stored material for medical students and residents, containing typical and/or interesting case reports, and images were available for all participants on the Internet (www.varimed.hu) [3,17].

Table 11.1. Statistical data of consultations (1 November 2001–16 July 2002 – BePro)	
Cases (total)	161
Image numbers (total)	786
Duration of consultations (case/min/mean)	13,18
Participating pathologists (department/case)	3
Average age of patients	52
Female	53
Male	49

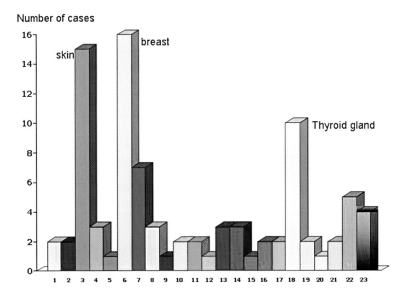

Fig. 11.3. Number and organ type of consulted cases. 1, brain; 2, intestine; 3, skin; 4, bone; 5, bone marrow; 6, breast; 7, stomach; 8, nerve; 9, soft tissue; 10, liver; 11, uterus; 12, parathyroid gland; 13, adrenal gland; 14, mesentery; 15, salivary gland; 16, lymph node; 17, ovary; 18, thyroid gland; 19, pancreas; 20, retroperitoneum; 21, oral cavity; 22, lung; 23, kidney

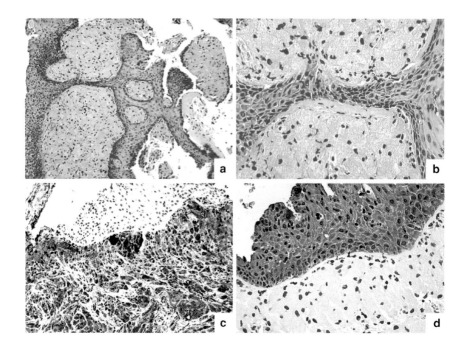

Fig. 11.4. Image archivation by DICOM, data transmission through XML data structures. (**a**) Histological image of the biopsy. Note squamous epithelium on the surface and tumor tissue in the deeper layers (HE, ×150). (**b**) The tumor cells possess abundant granular cytoplasm (HE, ×600). (**c**) The tumor cells show S100 positivity (S100 immunoperoxidase, ×300). (**d**) The tumor cells are negative for cytokeratine; epithelial cells show positivity (cytokeratine immunoperoxidase, ×600)

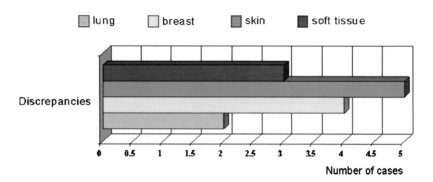

Fig. 11.5. Location and number of tumors where the second opinion modified the initial microscopic diagnosis

11.4.4
Main Results of the Bepro Project

The telepathology network established in the course of this project provided the basis for the application of telepathology integrated to a sophisticated informatics system. New standards such as DICOM, CEN TC251, etc., created by the European health-care telematics providers, were implemented in the network. The use of extended applied language (extensible markup language, XML) made possible the filling up, actualization, and harmonization of oncopathological databases, providing a platform for sharing professional practice information and results through the Internet and the regulation of data handling. XML developmental environment enabled the participating pathologists to actively contribute to web-based electronic protocols in their everyday practice. The system proved suitable for the transmission of macro- and microscopic images, including paraffin-embedded or frozen sections stained for routine histology or with special stains and cytological smears.

11.5
The Era of Digital Slides in Hungary

Based on previous experience and a fruitful cooperation between the Departments of Pathology of Semmelweis University, the MI Central Hospital, and a Hungarian spin-off company of digital microscopy (3DHISTECH Ltd., Budapest), since 2002, common efforts have been made to test the use of virtual slides for pathological purposes and share experiences with pathologists in the country. 3DHISTECH have produced automated Mirax slide scanners (www.3dhistech.com) distributed by Zeiss GmbH worldwide and developed software tools for pathological applications, including teleconsultation, teaching, and research, which have been tested and used in real situations by the partner pathology departments.

11.5.1
The Potential of Digital Slides in Histopathology

Availability of complete slides in digital/virtual format accessible, through the computer monitor by using dedicated software for easy navigation, to any part of the slide with arbitrary magnifications offered an unbeatable option for modernizing histopathology (Fig. 11.6). However, limitations of computer technology, including processor and network communication speed and storage capacity, were a real "bottleneck" up to the most recent years.

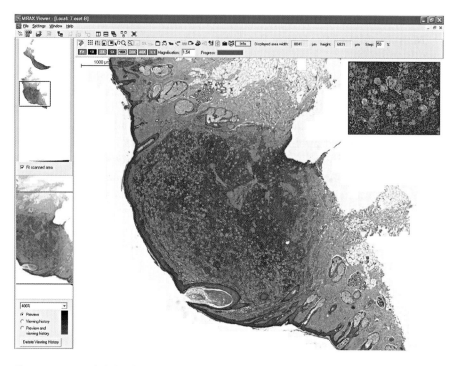

Fig. 11.6. Digital slide of an H&E-stained skin tumor revealed by using the Mirax Viewer software

During scanning of histology and cytology samples, digital slides are assembled from microscopic field of views (FOV), usually taken with a ×20 objective at a ~10 FOV/s speed and arranged at high precision along the X–Y coordinates [11]. They can be studied as image pyramids where low-power views are created by increasing compression of the original FOVs and using more and more of them at the same time, which ensures in-focus images at any magnification and sensible use of computer power. Scanning of fluorescing signals is also available for immunofluorescence and fluorescence in situ hybridization (FISH) [16]. By now, computer technology allows an average-sized 2–$3\,cm^2$ slide to be digitalized in transmission light mode in less than 8 min consisting of ~6,000 FOV to make up a 600 MB file, and up to 300 slides to be scanned in one run, which would nearly allow a medium-sized department to regularly archive all their diagnostic slides provided with proper informatics support [13].

Upgraded features of digital slides to traditional slides include easy annotations, fast and quality archiving of any field of interest at high color fidelity and even illumination, and simultaneous navigation and comparison of serial sections stained differently. In case of blood smears or FISH samples, Z-stacking of optical layers and the use of ×40 scanning objective ensures high resolution and/or small signals to be traced accurately. Serial digital slides can also be assembled into a three-dimensional structure for reconstructing the original tissue architecture. The discrete nature of information stored in pixels allows size and intensity measurements at high precision, opening up the avenue for automated image–object quantification, which can be of great importance in research and diagnostic histopathology, particularly in determining therapeutic targets [4,5].

Digital slides can be accessed by a number of pathologists through internal or external networks, and these can be integrated into existing digital databases of pathology reporting and archiving systems, which may also incorporate image archives of imaging diagnostic disciplines (X-rays, PET scans, etc.). Large slide archives can be created using the concept of slide archive and communication system (SACS).

Therefore, traditional slides do not lose importance in the era of digital slides, rather their information content can be fully exploited and made more easily accessible to pathologists in the form of digital slides.

11.5.2
Pilot Studies for Telepathology Using Digital Slides

Sharing digital slides through Intra- or Internet has a great potential in consulting difficult diagnostic cases and asking for a second opinion to improve diagnostic accuracy and exercise external quality assurance (EQA) of diagnostic activities.

One of the first studies evaluating the feasibility of virtual microscopy for diagnostic purposes using remote evaluation through the Internet was published by a Hungarian group, based on the cooperation between Semmelweis University and 3DHistech Ltd. [14]. Over 92% diagnostic concordance between virtual- and optical-microscopy-based evaluations of gastric biopsies already showed the potential of virtual microscopy, although scanning speed and transmission of digital slides were slow and image resolution was not suitable to reveal subtle structures, such as bacteria, that is, *Helicobacter pylori*.

Several other pilot studies followed, using upgraded virtual microscope software called Mirax Viewer and taking advantages of the improvements in scanning and computer technology. In a study presented at the ECP Congress in Paris (2005), accurate diagnosis could be established in 1,500 randomly selected cases of gastrointestinal, endocrine, soft tissue, and skin biopsies by using virtual and remote assessment through Intranet [19]. The most critical factors concluded were the same as for physical/optical slides, that is, section thickness and staining quality, which underlined the improvements in scanning technique and the importance of histotechnology as a key precondition for gaining appropriate digital image quality.

In another pilot study in 2006, relying on external teleconsultation through the Internet, over 100 randomly selected cases diagnosed locally using traditional microscopy were scanned and uploaded to server in the MI Central Hospital (Peter Gombas) to be diagnosed again at the second Department of Pathology at Semmelweis University (Gyorgy Illyes), using digital slides. Personal consultation revealed a 95% concordance between diagnoses, with no clinical consequences in the discordant cases.

11.6
Present and Future of Dynamic Telepathology in Hungary

It became obvious from the pilot studies that wide access to telepathology consultation services in the country requires substantial financial resources and educating pathologists. Slide scanners and software tools have to be deployed at the participating laboratories, and dedicated external server(s) need to be set up to minimize interference of huge image files with local firewalls [11].

An important step in spreading the idea of using digital slides and teleconsultation in Hungarian pathology was the establishment of www.pathonet.org portal by 3DHistech Ltd., with the cooperation of the Hungarian Society of Pathologists (Fig. 11.7). The website, professionally supervised by the College of Hungarian Pathologists, allows free access to digital slides incorporated into public cases, slide seminars, educational materials and e-books, and EQA.

Most importantly, a teleconsultation platform with appropriate software support is available, and assessment of digital slides can be done either online with the requesting pathologist or offline any time (Fig. 11.8). The demo version of Mirax Viewer software, allowing most microscopic functions accessible, can be downloaded and used freely. Users of the pathonet site need to register and can ask for storage space for uploading their digital slides if requesting teleconsultation or second opinion from either specialist using the website or any external experts. Since the limiting factor in exercising dynamic telepathology routinely is the lack of slide scanners at most institutes, the teleconsultation service is still in its pilot stage; however, besides Hungarian pathologists several foreign experts have tested the system.

Recently, the demand for a nationwide teleconsultation service in pathology has come from several directions. The legislation of confidential data protection in the course of nationwide telepathology consultations is established by Hungarian law on human rights (LXIII/1992 and XLVII/1997). Because of a controversial

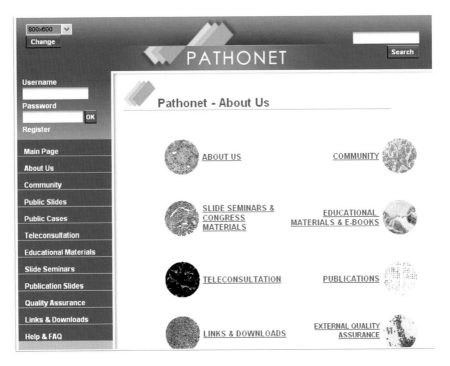

Fig. 11.7. The "pathonet" website, run by 3DHistech in cooperation with the Hungarian Society of Pathologists, offers a wide range of options for using digital slides in pathology

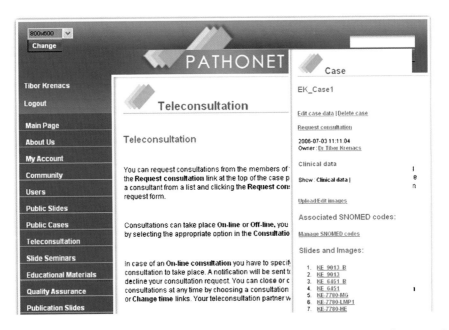

Fig. 11.8. The teleconsultation platform of the "pathonet" site. Uploaded cases with a range of clinicopathological data and digital slides are ready for teleconsultation on the sender's request

health-care reform in Hungary, a number of well-functioning hospital units have been closed; some hospitals in Budapest have been merged leaving numerous units without pathologists. On the contrary, the National Program for Cancer Prevention Program (2006) of the Hungarian Ministry of Health is aiming to modernize tumor diagnostics by supporting telepathology, which may contribute toward a more centralized, standardized, and cost-efficient diagnostic system. In line with these aims, financial resources were allocated in the Government Budget for 2006 for setting up a pilot network between a central institution and two remote pathology departments for testing teleconsultation in 1,000 diagnostic cases by the end of 2008. Unfortunately, this effort has also been delayed by the recent restrictive health-care reform.

So far, efforts for introducing telepathology have been driven by enthusiastic volunteer pathologists and have not been financed by any government body in Hungary. In accordance with this, the Hungarian Society of Pathology has most recently initiated and sent in an application for international grant support in association with 3DHistech Ltd. and Scandinavian partners, for setting up a regional/national teleconsultation network model system in Hungary, which can be adapted to any further regions in Europe and beyond. The aim of the project is to provide the instrumentation and software tools to all pathology institutions in Hungary and some Scandinavian partner institutions to test external communication and build up a network for routine diagnostic teleconsultations. Teleconsultation infrastructure could contribute to improving diagnostic accuracy in a time- and cost-efficient way, resulting in more accurate patient therapy. This facility would also improve the quality of gradual and postgradual teaching and would support life-long professional education and an upgraded EQA practice in the country.

11.6.1
Digital Microscopy for Teaching Histopathology in Hungary

11.6.1.1
E-Learning

The past decades have brought about substantial changes in higher education worldwide and in Hungary also. The amount and sophistication of information used in education, the expenses of university training, and number of students applying for admission to academic studies are gradually increasing. Teleeducation might be one answer to this socioeconomic challenge. The so-called virtual universities can supplement or replace theoretical trainings and contribute to practicals of today's universities. Virtual university, www.vu.org, has been one of the most traditional Internet-based learning communities since 1995, with over 2 million students from 128 countries attending its classes.

In the EU, several projects have aimed to develop communication technologies and adopt their achievements to e-learning. One of them was ACTS (1994–1998), Advanced Communications Technology and Services, as part of the "Fourth Framework Programme of European Community activities in the field of research and technological development and demonstration." The Final Report of ACTS initiated the building up of "virtual classrooms." In October 1995, students from the International School in Basel and the Glashan High School in Ottawa started working together, using ACTS broadband communications.

The main goals, expectations, and requirements of EU, Hungary as a new member state should meet in the field of e-learning, are concluded in the eEurope^{+2003} Action Plan (a cooperative effort to implement the information society in Europe), accepted by the EU Commission, in Goteborg, Sweden, 2001.

11.6.2
Digital Microscopy for Gradual Teaching

The medical qualification has always been a special field of education. As medics need to deal with human lives, there is no place for experimentation in the curricula and educational methods.

The staff of the first Department of Pathology and Experimental Cancer Research of Semmelweis University had collected many years of experience in virtual microscopy and run pilot digital histology courses before, as the first institution in Hungary, installed a virtual pathology laboratory, and started systematically using this facility for histopathology practicals in the 2007–2008 academic year (Fig. 11.9).

The system was successfully tested in 2006 in one of the computer laboratories of the Semmelweis University on histology practical courses for dentistry students [7]. Its workflow is similar to that of a teleconsultation. Every student has his/her own computer connected to a host, controlled by the teacher. The slide and its browsing by the consultant appear on the clients' monitors in real time. Students can disconnect from the consultation or request control over the slide to show challenging parts or structures to the teacher and to all the other students. Thus, instead of answering only for the student who finally dares to ask a question, the whole group can benefit from the answer. At the end of this pilot period, students were asked for their opinion on virtual microscopy (VM). On a 10-point scale, they gave an average of 8.7 score on how they liked the practice with VM. An average of 8.9 score was given when VM was compared to optical microscopy, and an average score of 8.8 was given for the user friendliness of VM. Finally, significantly more information was memorized with VM with OM.

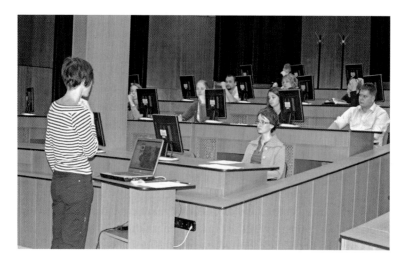

Fig. 11.9. Digital histopathology practice theatre in action. The facility was set up in 2007 at the first Department of Pathology and Experimental Cancer Research, Semmelweis University, Budapest

Based on positive feedback, virtual microscopes officially replaced their optical counterparts in pathology teaching from September 2007 in our department. The educational material provided to students is fully digitized and uploaded to the www.pathonet.org web portal. Through this site, students can revise the digital slides used in practicals and can more easily prepare for examinations.

11.6.3
Digital Microscopy for Postgradual Teaching, EQA, and E-Learning

The www.pathonet.org portal also provides storage space for digitized postgraduate educational material. Slides selected for scanning are from routine biopsy (rarely autopsy) archives of the past two decades, representing a broad spectrum of diseases from the most typical ones to real rarities. Altogether, over 500 digital slides are available for teaching pathology residents (Fig. 11.10).

Digital slides can be used in EQA programs [2]. In cooperation with national (QualiCont) and international (UK NEQAS ICC and NordiQC) EQA organizations, the pathonet portal is also used for uploading digital slides of assessment runs to demonstrate good and bad examples of staining quality, accompanied with critical notes and suggestions for improvement. Blood smears from the last three runs of the Hungarian Haematology EQA program organized by QualiCont are available digitally on the pathonet site for interpretation, in parallel

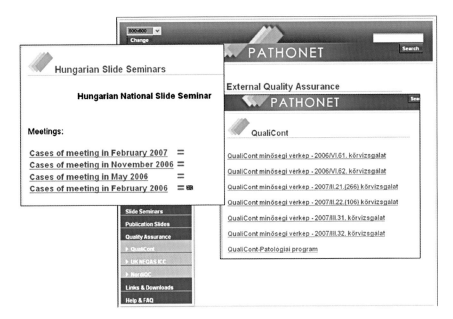

Fig. 11.10. Digital slide series of slide seminars held in Hungary in the last 2 years and digital blood smears uploaded for interpretation in the last three runs of the Haematology Quali-Cont EQA Program

with the physical smears for evaluating the efficiency of digital microscopy in hematology.

Recently, a teaching software-package, called E-School, was developed, which exploits the full potential of digital microscopy/pathology for publishing, producing educational material, practice/examination tests, and managing examinations accessible via the Internet for self-testing [8] (Fig. 11.11).

11.7
Video Conference Services for the Hungarian Higher-Education and Research Community

Video conferences offer a comprehensive way for interactive dispersal of knowledge in pathology where digital slides can also be included and projected. This facility can support postgraduate courses, slide seminars, and special lectures for medical students, resident, and pathologists all over the country (Fig. 11.12).

The first national initiative, called Information Infrastructure Development (IIF) program started in 1986, with the goal of establishing a computer network

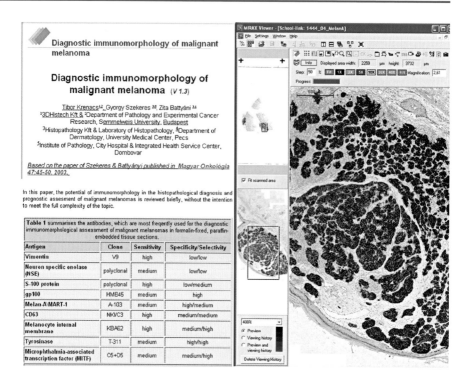

Fig. 11.11. An e-book on melanoma immunodiagnostics supplemented with linked digital slides and referred digital papers, freely accessible on www.pathonet.org

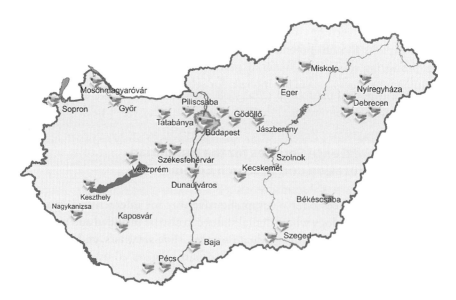

Fig. 11.12. NIF network in Hungary

(HBONE) for supporting research, higher education, and public collection communities in Hungary. In the early 1990s, the former IIF program was reorganized as the National Information Infrastructure Development (NIIF) program. In the last 20 years, development of NIIF network and its services has closely followed European progression of research networking by providing services from high-speed data networking to supercomputing and collaboration services.

NIIF program started its video conference service in late 2003. In the framework of the project, a country-wide ITU-T H.323 standard-based video conference network infrastructure and basic services were deployed. These include a high-capacity multipoint control unit (MCU) to host multipoint video conferences, a scalable gatekeeper network with interconnection to international IP-based video conference dialing services (GDS, global dialing scheme) and web-based end-user services. Today, NIIF video conference network offers various services to support multimedia collaboration: web based conference reservation system, information base, online statistics and automated video conference recording, and streaming facilities. They are provided mainly for member institutions and to support international research projects, free of charge.

11.8
Conclusion

During the past decades, enormous developments have taken place in telepathology worldwide and Hungarian professionals are very keen on catching up and taking part in modernizing of technology in pathology. Considering the most recent leaps in information technology and virtual microscopy, enormous developments are expected in the next 10 years toward the fully digitized support of pathology laboratories, where established tools of pathology will not lose importance, rather their information content will be easily accessed, controlled, measured, and shared with others.

11.9
Summary

The points discussed in the chapter can be summarized as follows:

- Historical background of telepathology in Hungary
- First steps to introduce telepathology in Hungary
- Development of telepathology in Hungary supported by the European Union

- Structure, function, and results of BePro
- The era of digital slides in Hungary
- Present stage and perspectives of virtual microscopy in Hungary
- Videoconference services for higher education and research in Hungary

References

1. Allen EA, Ollayos CW, Tellado MV, et al (2001) Characteristics of a telecytology consultation service. Human Pathol 32:1323–1326
2. Burthem J, Brereton M, Ardern J, et al (2005) The use of digital "virtual slides" in the quality assessment of hematological morphology: results of a pilot exercise involving UK NEQAS(H) participants. Br J Haematol 130:293–296
3. Cserneky M, Szende B, Vári S, et al (2002) Telepathology network in Hungary. Anal Cell Pathol 24(6):189
4. Ficsor L, Varga V, Berczi L, et al (2006) Automated virtual microscopy of gastric biopsies. Cytometry B Clin Cytom 70:423–431
5. Ficsor L, Varga VS, Jonas V, et al (2007) Validation of automated image analysis (HistoQuant) in colon cancer using digital slides of EGFR, Cox-2, beta-Catenin and CyclinD1 immunostainings. Virchows Arch 451:232
6. Fischer SI, Nandedkar MA, Williams BH, Abbondanzo L (2001) Telepathology in a clinical consultative practice. Human Pathol 32:1327–1333
7. Fonyad L (2006) Experience with building up a telepathology workstation and testing it for gradual education. 8th European Congress on Telepathology and 2nd International Congress on Virtual Microscopy, Budapest, July 6–8
8. Fonyad L, Zalatnai A, Ficsor L, Montvai M, Molnar B, Kopper L (2007) "I am still learning", introducing E.School, a new way to study pathology. Virchows Arch 451:583
9. Gombás P, Szende B, Stotz GY (1996) Future aspects and benefits of telematic networks used in pathology for countries of central Europe (CCE). Electron J Pathol Histol 963
10. Gombás P, Szende B, Stotz GY (1996) Support by telecommunication of decisions in diagnostic pathology. Experience with the first telepathology system in Hungary (in Hungarian with English abstract). Orvi Hetil 137:2299–2303
11. Gombás P, Skepper JN, Krenacs T, Molnar B, Hegyi L (2004) Past, present and future of digital pathology (in Hungarian with English Abstract). Orv Hetil 145:433–443
12. Kayser K, Fritz P, Drlicek M (1995) Aspects of telepathology in routinary diagnostic work with specific emphasis on ISDN. Arch Anat Cytol Pathol 43(4):216–218
13. Kayser K, Molnar B, Weinstein RS (2006) Virtual slide technology. In: Kayser K, Molnar B, Weinstein RS (eds) Virtual microscopy. Veterinarspiegel Verlag GmbH, Berlin, pp. 103–123
14. Molnar B, Berczi L, Diczhazy CS, et al (2003) Digital slide and virtual microscopy based routine and telepathology evaluation of routine gastrointestinal biopsy specimens. J Clin Pathol 56:433–438
15. Schwarzmann P, Schmid J, Schnorr C, Strassle G, Witte S (1995) Telemicroscopy stations for telepathology based on broadband and ISDN connections. Arch Anat Cytol Pathol 43(4):209–215

16. Varga VS, Ficsor L, Kamaras V, Molnar B, Tulassay ZS (2007) Automated fluorescent slide scanning. Virchows Arch 451:584

17. Vári S, Cserneky M, Kádár A, Szende B (2005) Development of present and future of telepathology in Hungary. Pathol Oncol Res 11(3):174–177

18. Weinstein RS, Descour MR, et al (2001) Telepathology overview: from concept to implementation. Human Pathol 23:1283–1299

19. Zalatnai A, Szende B, Berczi L, Fonyad L, Kopper L (2005) Working experience with digital slide and virtual microscopy-based routine and telepathology evaluation of biopsy specimens. Virchows Arch 447:516

Telecytology: A Retrospect and Prospect

Aruna Prayaga

12.1
Background Information

Cytology is a branch of pathology, with the main objective of delivering health care with rapidity and at a low cost. Cytopathologists, residents in pathology, fellows in cytology, cytotechnologists, and cytotechnicians are the people involved in the services. The study of the material involves screening and interpretation. Evaluation of cervicovaginal smears forms a major portion of the work, while most of the other material is obtained as fine-needle aspiration (FNA) or the effusion cytology. The samples received in the laboratory are first processed by the cytotechnicians. The cytotechnologists then screen the smears for cellular abnormalities and mark the areas of interest to be seen by the cytopathologists for all nongynecologic specimens and abnormal cervicovaginal specimens. Cytopathologists are responsible for the diagnosis of neoplastic lesions and all the difficult cases marked by the cytotechnologists.

Telecytology is remote consultation on the cytologic smears using digital images and is similar to telepathology (Fig. 12.1). However, it has a few special requirements.

How does telecytology differ from telepathology?

- Imaging of larger area and more number of images for determination of adequacy and diagnosis
- Require higher magnification and more color depth
- Limited and perishable material
- Relative lack of pattern
- Three-dimensional cell clusters
- Additional category of health-care personnel: cytotechnologists

Conventional cytologic smears occupy more area on the glass slide than the histopathologic material. Hence, screening and imaging the entire glass slide is more tedious. Lower-magnification images cover more area of the glass slide but lack resolution and are blurred [25]. Determination of adequacy and assessment

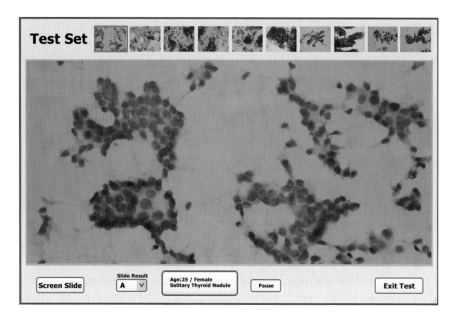

Fig. 12.1. A module with images for telecytology, thumb nails and magnified, stained with Papanicolaou and May–Grunwald Giemsa (MGG) stains

of cellularity are important requirements in cytology samples, as a few atypical cells in poorly cellular samples need to be interpreted with caution. The tendency for the person capturing the images is to focus on the cellular areas. So there is a possibility of a false assessment of adequacy. Material obtained for histopathologic examination are preserved as paraffin blocks. It is possible to cut these blocks to obtain the tissue for consultation or as teaching material. In telepathology practice, a few low-magnification images can indicate alteration in pattern in the tissue sections, and higher-magnification images from those areas may be enough to make the diagnosis. Cytologic material is generally scant, most of which is smeared onto the glass slides; hence results in loss of tissue architecture, although individual cell morphology is excellently preserved. The glass slides can neither be transported easily nor be replicated. In addition, Papanicolaou stain is the basic cytologic stain with a range of colors to bring about the finer nuclear details like chromatin pattern, nuclear membrane irregularities, and cytoplasmic maturation. Colors must be reproduced accurately in the images for telecytology for proper interpretation. Higher magnification and better resolution are needed to examine chromatin texture and other finer details important for cytologic diagnosis. While histologic sections are cut with a certain thickness, cytology samples are smeared. Depending on the yield of the material, the smears may be scanty or thick. A cellular aspirate with tight clusters or hemorrhagic aspirate may form three-dimensional clusters. Focusing on the cells through these clusters is a special requirement for cytologic samples. Screening of cervicovaginal smears requires trained cytotechnologists. Telecytology has a role to play in training and conducting proficiency testing for cytotechnologists and cytopathologists. Over the years it was realized that the advantages of telecytology sometimes outnumber those of telepathology. Despite these facts, cytologists around the world are hesitant to practise telecytology, as evidenced by fewer numbers of publications.

Possible reasons for resistance from the cytologists:

- Technophobia
- Lack of personal interaction with the patient
- Scant clinical and radiologic information
- Quality and adequacy of images
- Interaction between the person at the remote center and the consultant

As compared to telepathology, telecytology started a decade later and is still in its infancy. In a sample survey conducted in 1993, only four out of 166 members of the International Academy of Cytologists felt that telecytology had a diagnostic potential [30]. The survey highlighted the apprehensions of the members to use new technology. Most cytologists perform the FNAs themselves, giving them an opportunity to examine the patient, lesion, and the nature of the aspirate to form a preliminary opinion. However, this is not possible in telecytology practice. The number of images required to determine adequacy and for diagnosis is more. Hence, it is cumbersome for the person capturing the images and also for the person evaluating them. These issues are compounded by the general apprehension in telepathology practice about the quality of pictures, field selection, adequacy of the number of fields, limited access to clinical information, radiologic findings, and immunochemistry.

Initial studies have focused on testing the efficacy of this branch of telemedicine on cervicovaginal smears. Earliest documented study was by Calvert et al. who analyzed 40 cervicovaginal smears by transmitting the static images to five pathologists from a remote site [4]. Raab et al. have shown video images of dotted areas with a fixed, short viewing time for proficiency testing [23]. Videomicroscopy was used by Ziol et al. as well, and Alli et al. used digital images [34, 2].

At the Annual Conference of International Academy of Cytologists at Hawaii in 1997, an expert committee on "digital imagery/telecytology" discussed the role of telecytology for consultation, primary diagnosis, validation of diagnoses, and quality assurance [20]. They have also suggested that the scope can be extended to determine sample adequacy in image-guided aspirations, where the pathologist, sitting in his or her office, could confirm the adequacy of the material obtained by the procedure conducted by the radiologist. The committee reviewed various publications in the literature and concluded that there is a need to focus on the innovative methods to improve accuracy of telecytology.

12.2
Global Experience

Mairinger and Gschwendtner have cautioned against the use of limited static images and suggested that it can be the dead end for telecytology [17]. In doing so, they have quoted Leopold Koss, the father of modern cytology, who in his famous statement said that cytology is not mere study of the morphology of cells, it is the clinical context in which the cells are, and the entire specimen has to be examined for a meaningful conclusion, as the cytologic diagnosis is more difficult than histologic diagnosis.

In later years, telecytology using static images was extended to nongynecologic cytology [3,5,6,9]. Briscoe et al. studied 25 breast aspirates initially sent for second opinion with static images on limited selected fields with a good concordance. But the observers were less confident of their telecytologic diagnoses than of their glass slide diagnoses. At the same time, overdiagnoses outnumbered underdiagnoses. Hence, the authors emphasized the role of adequate information on clinical examination and mammography for better interpretation of the cytologic findings and suggested that refinement in the diagnostic criteria of malignancy is needed for better telecytologic interpretation [3].

Advantages of telecytology:

- Primary consultation
- Consultation for second opinion
- Shorter turnaround time for consultation
- Quality control
- Training of the cytotechnologists and residents
- Proficiency testing
- Documentation of data
- Testing adequacy of a procedure from a remote center

Allen et al. [1] studied the clinical usefulness of telecytology, concordance with the original or the glass slide diagnosis, and the influence of image quality on the diagnosis. Both under- and overdiagnoses were observed on telecytology when compared with the glass slides. There was concordance between telecytologic and glass slide diagnosis in 69% of the cases, and the discordance seen in rest of the cases was minor. Diagnosis was deferred in one case due to poor staining, out-of-focus images, and scant cellularity. In the second case, diagnosis was made subsequently with better images. The authors expressed their satisfaction with the existing technology, for imaging and transferring technology are not the limiting factors for the practice of telecytology. Diagnostic accuracy and the confidence with which the diagnosis was made were not affected by the image format, resolution, or method of transmission. Although it was mandatory to review glass slides as a quality assurance method, only 26% of the cases received glass slides. The contributing pathologists might have feared breakage, loss, or nonreturn of the slides. The authors reviewed the literature and concluded that the concordance with glass slides is better for telepathology than for telecytology.

Yamashiro et al. [33] published the largest number of routine cases subjected for telecytology from Hokkaido island of Japan to Sapporo National Hospital. Majority of the images were with 40× magnification. The results were highly encouraging, with κ value of 0.919 for cervical smears and 0.810 for specimens other than cervical smears. They have observed that the reasons for incorrect diagnoses were similar to conventional cytologic diagnoses and lack of familiarity with the lesions. Moreover, there was a tendency to be definitive in telecytology probably due to psychological factors. The authors emphasized the importance of good communication and frank discussions of cytologic and clinical findings between the cytologists and cytotechnologists. Efficient operation of digital camera and computer network are important requirements but are less important compared with the diagnostic skills of the participants and their professional relationships. Many participants who viewed the images and followed the e-mail discussions helped them to reappraise the diagnoses in a few cases [13].

Marchevsky et al. [18] compared the results of four experienced cytopathologists in telecytology and conventional microscopy of well-differentiated adenocarcinoma and chronic pancreatitis with atypical epithelial changes due to repair. The authors used 100× magnification and zoomed the images 8×. To their surprise, they found that the telecytology results correlated better with the original diagnosis than the conventional microscopy. They concluded that it was probably because the virtual slides were faster and easier to examine, as the consultants had to review relatively smaller number of preselected fields for examination. Moreover, larger images than microscopy by zooming provided better appreciation of the subtle features like membrane irregularity and irregular chromatin clumping. Telecytology thereby provides an opportunity to seek expert opinion in difficult areas of cytology.

In veterinary practice, telecytology starts from the consultation rooms, enabling the physicians to telescope the time for evaluation and faster delivery of health care [10,31]. Allen et al. [1] also opined that the major advantage of telecytology in the daily workflow is the shorter time taken for teleconsultation compared with conventional method of sending the glass slides by ordinary mail.

Computerized testing is in use for certification of the cytotechnologists in the United States of America, but, for training and proficiency testing, manual screening of the glass slides is still the gold standard. An International Expert Committee on Computerized Training and Proficiency Testing has made a few recommendations [29]:

- Computerized training should be able to identify submarginal performers early.
- Training programs should emphasize the differences between digital images and light microscopic features.
- There should be interactive capability allowing educational feedback.
- It is necessary to have devices to aid in automatic screening of the entire slide, recording the information, and recalling the areas marked by the screener.
- For proficiency testing, the system should be able to test both screening and diagnostic abilities.

The advantages of computer training and proficiency testing as seen by the committee are the following:

- Integration of multiple fields in a single montage
- Ready duplication and transportation
- Availability of standardized teaching sets
- Standardization of terminology and criteria can be facilitated as they have wider reach
- Could ease burden on teaching staff
- Training can be tailored to individual capabilities

Training in cytology includes the training of the cytotechnologists, postgraduates, and fellows. These groups can use telecytology for learning at their pace. Cytotechnologists can be trained to select suspicious areas for screening by the cytopathologists. Limited and preselected images are useful in proficiency testing and quality control. Proficiency testing can be done periodically for all the practitioners of cytology, which is otherwise not possible because of organizational problems involved [16,19]. Lee et al. have studied the role of digital images in cervicovaginal cytology for quality assurance. In laboratories where quality assurance exercises are frequent and several laboratories are involved in the program, it is difficult to circulate the glass slides as the turnaround time of glass slides is slow; several participants had to attend the meetings without a chance to see the slides. To overcome this problem, the authors have posted preselected, digitized images on the website. As a result, the turnaround time was reduced to half. The images ensured assessment of identical fields, and the aim of the program was to test the ability of the participants to make correct diagnosis and not the ability to screen the slides. The authors could also save time and money, as they did not have to mail the glass slides. Telecytologic experience in addition to cytologic experience is essential to improve diagnostic accuracy [6].

Gagnon et al. [8] have explored the utility of computer-based proficiency testing for a group of 111 cytopathologists and cytotechnologists. The software used was capable of stitching more than 8,000 images together digitally and could also change the focal plane. In spite of this, the candidates fared poorly with virtual slides than with the glass slides. The authors suggested that with proper field validation of virtual images, telecytology could replace glass slides for proficiency testing. In a study conducted by Stewart et al. [26], three cytotechnologists marked the diagnostic areas on virtual slides of liquid-based cytology preparations. The study proved the role of virtual microscopy in cytotechnology education to evaluate the ability of the student to locate the abnormal cells and diagnose.

Most of the studies showed acceptable to near-perfect kappa values of telecytologic results compared with the glass slides and between the observers. In samples with limited diagnostic possibilities, the accuracy is higher. Yamashiro et al. encountered less than acceptable results in biliary cytology [33]. Inadequate and improper sampling is the common reason for low diagnostic accuracy. A close interaction with the cytotechnologist at the remote center and the telecytologist is mandatory for meaningful teleconsultation for a primary diagnosis. Similar understanding is necessary between the expert and the cytologist seeking the opinion for second opinion as well.

12.3
Future Perspective

Utility of telecytology has been validated in primary consultation, second opinion, training, proficiency testing, and certification. Issues that need to be addressed are the following:

- Amalgamating newer technologies for sample processing and for improvement of images
- Incorporation of images into the patients' files
- Off-site assessment of adequacy in guided aspirations and endoscopic procedures
- Legal issues
- Redefining morphologic criteria suitable for telecytologic practice
- Recruiting more number of cytologists into telecytology

Limited, preselected static imaging is slowly paving way for automated complete slide digitization. Entire slide can be scanned at all the magnifications available in the microscope, and the cytopathologists can view the images on the computer screen. The images can be magnified, and the area of interest can be zoomed without loss of resolution. These images are much bigger than the microscopic fields. These virtual slides are very large and need to be stored in virtual slide boxes.

In conventional cytology practice, changing the focal plane helps the cytologist to examine the cells in three-dimensional clusters. Ability of an imaging system to change the focus is referred to as z-axis imaging. In "store-and-send" static image method of telecytology, this is not possible. Robotic systems allow real-time examination of the slide; the operator from a remote center can change the field and the focus. Utility of the robotic system is challenged by the prohibitive cost. Automated slide digitization is done by imaging at different focal planes and superimposing them in a three-dimensional image tile.

Liquid-based cytology has originally started for automated screening of cytologic smears and gained popularity for routine manual screening. As the smears made by liquid-based cytology are in a limited area and in monolayered sheets, it is easier to scan these and focus the cells, and hence it can be very useful in the practice of telecytology. Relatively clean background seen with these smears improves the clarity. Kaplan et al. [12] studied 80 consecutive abnormal thin prep pap smears using remote-controlled microscope. Interestingly, all the four glandular lesions could not be interpreted because groups of glandular cells could not be focused and the diagnosis was deferred. There were four discrepant cases where the diagnosis of the cytotechnologist on glass slide was atypical squamous cells of undetermined significance (ASCUS) and the telecytologic diagnosis was negative for intraepithelial lesion (NIL). Subsequent review and serologic tests for human papillomavirus (HPV) proved that interpretation based on telecytology to be more accurate. Hence, the practice of liquid-based cytology should be encouraged as it can contribute to better images.

Eichhorn et al. [7] suggested a model for cervical smear screening in the developing countries. One objective of the study was to triage the patients into high- and low-risk groups for carcinoma. Smears prepared by liquid-based cytology were screened by an automated screening system, which was capable of capturing low-resolution, black and white images. Thirty-two cases with wide range of cytologic diagnoses were selected, and the images were sent by e-mail to two cytopathologists at the "reading station" for interpretation. The patients were categorized into two categories: one was negative for malignancy and low-grade lesions and second one was high grade and more serious process. The pathologists viewed the images twice to find out whether there could be improvement in interpretation with experience considering the quality of images. After the first evaluation, the interpretation results were compared with the original diagnosis. Two months later, the images were reshuffled for reinterpretation. There was an overall concordance rate of 84%, with a sensitivity of 63% and specificity of 92% for both the trials. One pathologist improved on sensitivity and the other on specificity. The authors hypothesized that in the developing countries, where there is shortage of trained workforce, this model will be helpful for population-based screening. They highlighted a few morphologic features that are relatively unaffected by the quality of images, including nuclear cytoplasmic ratio, nuclear shape, degree of hyperchromasia, cellular relations in the aggregates, and HPV-associated cytopathic perinuclear vacuoles. Background features like inflammation and tumor diathesis were useful in the diagnosis.

Reproducibility of colors is important in pathology and more so in cytology. In the studies published so far, with the available digital cameras, resolution and representation of color appear adequate, and improper representation of color has not been highlighted as a major problem. The future technologies may also address the issue of improving the currently available 24-bit colors.

Incorporation of the images in patients' files will enable them to get treated anywhere in the world by the expert of his or her choice. Stewart et al. used picture archival and communication system (PACS) to digitally acquire static images and incorporated them into the patients' reports with digital imaging and communication in medicine (DICOM) format. Based on a written survey of the clinicians, the authors concluded that this will immensely help in the exchange of diagnostic information and improve the patient care [27]. As mentioned earlier, cytologic material is available in the form of glass slides which are perishable. Hence, the virtual slide used in telecytology can be used for external and internal quality control. They can be sent to the sponsors for evaluation during clinical trials.

Another potential utility is to determine adequacy in guided aspirations. FNA cytology of deep-seated lesions is done under imageologic guidance. Diagnostic accuracy of computed tomography (CT)- and endoscopic ultrasound (EUS)-guided aspirations depends on adequacy of the material obtained. Cost of these procedures is high and requires on-site determination of adequacy by a cytologist or cytotechnologists, demanding significant amount of their time. If the slide can be focused in the radiology department and the pathologist can view it under the microscope in his/her office, it will save a lot of time [27]. In a double-blind study on telediagnosis of transbronchial fine-needle aspirate, Kayser et al. found total agreement between telecytologic and conventional diagnoses in differentiating benign lesions from malignant lesions and also small-cell carcinoma from nonsmall-cell carcinoma. They have recommended the use of telecytology during endoscopy to avoid repeat procedure in the event of a nonproductive aspiration [14]. Kim et al. conducted a similar study in pancreatic carcinomas [15].

The feasibility of robotic telecytology in a case of endoscopic ultrasound-guided FNA (EUS-FNA) was studied by Robbins et al., and the difficulties encountered compared with static images were discussed. Robotic screening produced movement artifacts, and focusing was slower. However, the authors opined that with minor refinements, robotic telecytology could expand the link between the endoscopist and the cytologist [24].

Oberholzer from the department of Pathology of the University Hospital Basel, Switzerland, has started an e-group, iPath, a user-friendly Linux-based system. The members are divided into two groups: nonexperts and experts. Nonexperts deposit a question or a problem with clinical details, images, and comments. The experts answer the questions. The authors feel that iPath will help in globalization of cytology [21].

Briscoe et al. [3] have suggested refinement in the morphologic criteria used for the diagnosis of malignancy, considering the advantages and limitations of telecytology systems. It is also necessary to use uniform terms for diagnosis. Classifying the lesions of individual organs numerically does not have wide acceptance as it has limitations. But if we have to use telecytology routinely, it will be prudent to accept numerical system of classification, retaining the opportunity to individualize the case. Adding the images of radiographic and clinical photographs and results of immunocytochemistry can enhance the diagnostic accuracy.

The Expert Committee on digital imagery grouped legal issues into three categories [20]:

- Licensing of telecytologists
- Confidentiality and informed consent
- Malpractice liability

These above issues are practitioner related; technical aspects include the image resolution and color characteristics [2]. In addition, specification and updation of the equipment also need to be included. Japanese government addressed the issue based on the type of the system used. Responsibility rests with the consultant if the system used is robotic microscope at the remote site. In the passive diagnostic system, the person at the remote center by whom the images have been selected and transmitted will be responsible [28].

12.3.1
Indian Scenario

Most of the telecytologic consultation in India is for second opinion and the studies conducted are pilot studies [11,22]. Several pathologists use Internet services to consult an expert at a personal level. Members participating in cytology group of http://iPath.ch are fewer compared with the pathology group. Legal issues have not been addressed so far, as the primary pathologist has the choice to accept or ignore the opinion of the expert.

The only live study was from Tata Memorial Hospital, Mumbai. Jialdasani et al. studied 46 cytology smears from a remote center in 2 years. A comparison was made between the telepathology and telecytology services. The authors needed double the number of images for telecytology. Relative lack of pattern was another disadvantage. During the telepathology consultations, the authors were able to insist on the area of interest in lower magnification. However, in telecytology consultation, the authors had to depend entirely on the images sent by referring pathologist [11].

In India, there are more than 1,500 pathologists practicing cytology. However, qualified cytotechnologists are only around 150. Majority of the cytotechnologists are in the urban areas and with the leading cancer centers. Barring these centers, there is no separate category of cytotechnologists in the employment market of the country, and they are treated on par with the rest of the technologists. The number of the cytotechnologists must increase to man the remote centers, to capture the images, and to send them to the consultant. Liquid-based cytology has not found its place in India yet. Utility of cytopathology with "store-and-send" images for primary diagnosis in this situation is questionable. However, it may be added that the processing of material for cytologic evaluation is simple compared to the processing required for histopathology. If the health-care personnel at the remote centers can be trained to image the entire slide with newer systems, telecytology can be used for primary consultation. In this context, telecytology linked with liquid-based cytology and automated screening can be useful. Cytotechnologists may be pooled in a few centers for manual review of the images [7]. This can also give them an advantage of consulting and learning from each other.

Availability of funds for the software and hardware was a limiting factor. With rapid advancement in information technology in India, it is now possible to transmit images with greater ease. Government of India, is showing keen interest in telemedicine. Indian Space Research Organization (ISRO) and several other organizations dealing with information technology are actively supporting the program with technical assistance. A few national conferences were conducted.

12.4
Education and Training Opportunities Available

1. http://telemed.ipath.ch/ipath; accessed on 14 October 2007
2. http://teleteach.patho.unibas.ch; accessed on 14 October 2007
3. http://www.vdic.com/telemedicine/telecytology.html; accessed on 14 October 2007

Telecytology has come a long way from what was thought to be a dead end. Globalization of cytology is now possible, and the patient can choose to consult the physician of his/her choice from any corner of the world. There is a need to redefine the cytologic criteria for an effective use of telecytology, and with consistent efforts, diagnostic accuracy can be on par with conventional cytology. As the technologic advances are rapid, if cytologists around the world shed their resistance and accept telecytology as an alternative to conventional cytology, it may not be preposterous to think of "discarding the microscopes" [32].

12.5
Summary

- Telecytology is remote consultation on the cytologic smears using digital images and is similar to telepathology.
- Advantages of telecytology include primary consultation, consultation for second opinion, shorter turnaround time for consultation, quality control, training of the cytotechnologists and residents, proficiency testing, documentation of data, and testing adequacy of a procedure from a remote center.
- Issues that need to be addressed in telecytology include amalgamating newer technologies for improvement in images, incorporation of images into the patients' files, off-site assessment of adequacy in guided aspirations and endoscopic procedures, legal issues, redefining morphologic criteria suitable for telecytologic practice, and recruiting more number of cytologists into telecytology.
- Liquid-based cytology has originally started for automated screening of cytologic smears. As the smears made by liquid-based cytology are easier to be scanned, these can be very useful in the practice of telecytology.
- Telecytology has come a long way since its conception. Globalization of cytology is now possible, and the patient can choose to consult the physician of his/her choice from any corner of the world.

Acknowledgments

The author thanks Dr Rachel Thomas Jacob, Associate Professor, Nizam's Institute of Medical Sciences, for editing the manuscript.

References

1. Allen EA, Ollayos CW, Tellado MV, et al. (2001) Characteristics of a telecytology consultation service. Hum Pathol 32:1323–1326
2. Alli PM, Ollayos CW, Thomson LD, et al. (2001) Telecytology: intraobserver and interobserver reproducibility in the diagnosis of cervical-vaginal smears. Hum Pathol 32:1318–1322

3. Briscoe D, Adair CF, Thompson LD, et al. (2000) Telecytologic diagnosis of breast fine needle aspiration biopsies – intraobserver concordance. Acta Cytol 44:175–180
4. Calvert S, Mc Ginnis K, O'Dell D, Prey M, Odnault T, Skolom J (1994) Pap smear interpretation using computer imaging: an interlaboratory model (abstr). Am J Clin Pathol 102:537–538
5. da Silva VD, Prolla JC, Diehl AR, Baldo MF, Muller RL (1997) Comparison of conventional microscopy and digitized imaging for serous effusions. Anal Quant Cytol Histol 19:202–206
6. Della Mea V, Puglisi F, Bonzanini M, et al. (1997) Fine-needle aspiration cytology of the breast – a preliminary report on telepathology through Internet multimedia electronic mail. Mod Pathol 10:636–641
7. Eichhorn JH, Brauns TA, Geifand JA, Crothers BA, Wilbur DC (2005) A novel automated screening and interpretation process for cervical cytology using internet transmission of low-resolution images – a feasibility study. Cancer Cytopathol 105:199–206
8. Gagnon M, Inborn S, Hancock J, et al. (2004) Comparison of proficiency testing: glass slides vs. virtual slides. Acta Cytol 48:787–794
9. Glavez J, Howell L, Costa MJ, Davis R (1998) Diagnostic concordance of telecytology and conventional cytology for evaluating breast aspirates. Acta Cytol 42:663–667
10. Herbert P, Latouche JS, Menard M, Papageorges M (2001) Telecytology. Clin Tech Small Anim Pract 16:122–124
11. Jialdasani R, Desai S, Gupta M, et al. (2006) An analysis of 46 static telecytology cases over a period of two years. J Telemed Telecare 12:311–314
12. Kaplan KJ, Boast DL, Bolger AY (2004) Are current image resolutions sufficient for telecytology? ASC Bull 41:42–44
13. Kawamura N, Yamashiro K, Matsubayashi S, et al. (2004) Diagnostic results and its problems of telecytology utilizing internet. J Jpn Soc Clin Cytol 43:205–213
14. Kayser K, Kayser G, Becker HD, Herth F (2000) Telediagnosis of transbronchial fine needle aspirations – a feasibility study. Anal Cell Pathol 21:207–212
15. Kim B, Chhieng D, Jhala N, et al. (2006) Dynamic telepathology has equivalent efficiency with on site rapid cytology diagnoses for pancreatic carcinoma (abstract). Cancer Cytopathol 108S:357
16. Lee ES, Kim IS, Choi JS, et al. (2003) Accuracy and reproducibility of telecytology diagnosis of cervical smears. A tool for quality assurance programs. Am J Clin Pathol 119:356–360
17. Mairinger T, Gschwendtner A (1997) Telecytology using preselected fields of view: the future of cytodiagnosis or a dead end? Am J Clin Pathol 107:620
18. Marchevsky AM, Nelson V, Martin SE, et al. (2003) Telecytology of fine-needle aspiration biopsies of the pancreas: a study of well-differentiated adenocarcinoma and chronic pancreatitis with atypical epithelial repair changes. Diagn Cytopathol 28:147–152
19. Marchevsky AM, Wan Y, Thomas P, Krishnan L, Evan-Simon H, Haber H (2003) Virtual microscopy as a tool for proficiency testing in cytopathology: a model using multiple digital images of Papanicolaou tests. Arch Pathol Lab Med 127:1320–1324
20. O'Brien MJ, Takahashi M, Brugal G, et al. (1998) Digital imagery/telecytology. IAC Task Force Summary. Acta Cytol 42:148–164
21. Oberholzer (2007) Telecytology: a new path to globalisation of cytology (abstract). e-health/e-sante, accessed on October 14, 2007
22. Prayaga AK, Loya AC, Satish Rao I (2006) Telecytology – are we ready. J Telemed Telecare 12:319–320
23. Raab SS, Zaleski S, Thomas PA, Niemann TH, Isacson C, Jensen CS (1996) Telecytology: diagnostic accuracy in cervical–vaginal smears. Am J Clin Pathol 105:599–603

24. Robbins D, Rorat E, Sheridan G, Bodenheimer H, Wening B (2006) Robotic telecytology and EUS-FNA (abstract). Endoscopy 38; DOI:10.1055/s-2006-947776, accessed on October 7, 2008
25. Schwarzmann P, Schenck U, Binder B, Schmid J (1998) Is today's telepathology equipment also appropriate for telecytology? A pilot study with pap and blood smears. Adv Clin Pathol 2:176–178
26. Stewart J, Bevans-Wilkins K, Ye C, Miyazaki K, Kurtycz DFI (2006) Virtual microscopy: an educator tool for the enhancement of cytotechnology students' locator skills (abstract). Cancer Cytopathol 108S:445–446
27. Stewart J, Duncan LD, Li YJ, et al. (2006) Cost/benefit analysis of incorporating static digital images of cytopathology cases into picture archiving and communication system (abstract). Cancer Cytopathol 108S:346
28. Tsuchihashi Y, Okada Y, Ogushi Y, Mazaki T, Tsutsumi Y, Sawai T (2000) The current status of medicolegal issues surrounding telepathology and telecytology in Japan. J Telemed Telecare 6(Suppl 1):S143–S154
29. Vooijs GP, Davey DD, Somrak TM, et al. (1998) Computerized training and proficiency testing: IAC task force summary. Acta Cytol. 42:141–147
30. Wied GL (1994) The inevitable and mandatory computerization of our laboratories. In: Wied GL, Bartels PH, Rosenthal DL, Schenck U (eds) Compendium on computerized cytology and histology laboratory. Tutorials of Cytology, Chicago, pp. 11–12
31. William BH (2007) Telecytology – improving your practice with "micro management" www.afip.org/ferrets/PDF/telecytology.pdf. Accessed on October 5
32. Wojcik E (2004) Virtual microscopy – is it time to discard our microscopes? ASC Bull 41:37–41
33. Yamashiro K, Kawamura N, Matsatoshi S, et al. (2004) Telecytology in Hokkaido Island, Japan: results of primary telecytodiagnosis of routine cases. Cytopathology 15:221–227
34. Ziol M, Vacher-Lavenu MC, Heudes D, et al. (1999) Expert consultation for cervical smears. Reliability of selected field videomicroscopy. Anal Quant Cytol Histol 21:35–41

Teledermatopathology: Current Status and Perspectives

Cesare Massone, Alexandra Maria Giovanna Brunasso, and H. Peter Soyer

13.1
Introduction

Teledermatopathology allows remote diagnosis of skin specimens at remote locations by using computer and communications technology, and it can be performed with real-time (dynamic) transmission of images or the store-and-forward (SAF; static) option [3,16,23]. The first method provides remote consultation via a robotic microscope, which can be controlled by the consulting pathologist [3,16,23]. On the contrary, using the SAF system, each image is captured and transmitted as a single file. The fields to be examined are selected by the referring pathologist and then transmitted by an e-mail or a file transfer protocol (FTP) connection or using a specific web application [3,16,23]. In the last several years, virtual slide systems (VSSs) have been introduced in telepathology. With these systems, the whole slide can be digitized at high resolutions, which allows the user to view any part of the specimen at any magnification [8]. In this way, the limitations imposed by capturing small preselected areas can be overcome. Moreover, the acquired images can be stored on a virtual slide (VS) server that makes them available on the web, and an integrated VS client enables the users to browse the VS [8,23]. Recently, new ultrarapid VS processors have been developed [24].

In dermatopathology, the knowledge of skin physiology and semiotics should always be integrated with a clinical background to arrive at a correct diagnosis. The study of histopathologic specimens from inflammatory skin diseases and equivocal melanocytic lesions can be particularly difficult, and a strict correlation with clinical parameters becomes mandatory. Two examples of dermatopathologic entities that might be problematic in routine dermatopathology are inflammatory dermatoses, characterized by subtle pattern arrangements of inflammatory cells and dysplastic nevi, where subtle changes in architectural and cytologic appearance can lead astray to a more malignant behavior.

This issue is of major concern for achieving correct diagnoses in teledermatopathology [2, 16, 18]. The feasibility of both SAF and real-time teledermatopathology has already been proved in few studies, mainly on nonmelanoma skin cancer or melanocytic lesions, with less emphasis on inflammatory skin diseases [1, 2, 4, 6, 7, 16–19, 22]. These studies suggest that diagnostic efficacy and accuracy in teledermatopathology may be particularly weak when examining entities that require the identification of subtle architectural arrangements or delicate cytologic features, as in inflammatory skin diseases [1, 2, 4, 6, 7, 16–19, 22]. Recent applications of VSS in teledermatopathology both on melanocytic lesions and on inflammatory skin diseases confirmed the intrinsic difficulty of dermatopathology and teledermatopathology [11, 15]. Further development of the VSS and new studies using the new VS processor, as well as training with the virtual microscope, might improve the diagnostic performance of teleconsultants.

13.2
SAF Teledermatopathology

SAF-system is the most common application used in teledermatopathology. Each image is captured by a conventional camera/video camera adapted on a normal microscope. Images are saved on a smart card and then downloaded on a personal computer where editing can be done using image-specific software (i.e., Photoshop, Adobe Systems GmbH, Saggart, and Republic of Ireland). Then transmission as a single file through an e-mail or FTP to one or more teleconsultants can be done. During the transmission process, problems due to large image size can be easily solved by compressing the files using the joint photographic experts group (JPEG), which is the current standard compression format. In this way, images are then saved on the teleconsultant's personal computer and become not accessible for other teleconsultants. To seek further opinions on the same case, images need to be sent out again [2, 16, 18]. A recently introduced new option in SAF teledermatopathology consists in the use of specific web applications suited for teledermatopathology (i.e., http://telederm.org/research/dermatopath/default.asp) [11, 14, 15, 20]. With this system, images are uploaded and saved on the server of the specific web application. The advantage of this application relies on saving time; the avoidance of the compression phase allows the uploading of original files, which become immediately available to different teleconsultants simultaneously. The security and privacy of this web application are guaranteed by a personal login and password used by each teleconsultant to access the patients' data [11, 14, 15, 20].

The demonstration of SAF teledermatopathology and its feasibility have been proven in few studies, mainly on nonmelanoma skin cancer or on melanocytic lesions, with less emphasis on inflammatory skin diseases [1, 2, 4, 6, 7, 16–19, 22]. Weinstein et al. found 100% concordance of diagnosis and margin assessment in a retrospective study that involved a surgical pathologist and frozen-section analysis of mostly nonmelanoma skin cancer [22]. Similar results were obtained by Dawson et al. in the frozen-section assessment of resection margins for cutaneous basal-cell and squamous-cell carcinoma [4]. Della Mea et al. determined a κ statistic of 0.79 between two pathologists in a study of 20 melanocytic lesions [6]. Piccolo et al. showed a telepathology concordance rate of 78%, which improved to 85% with conventional microscopy in a series that involved 20 various dermatologic entities [19]. Okada et al. found a 100% concordance in a study of 35 melanocytic lesions between a general pathologist and a dermatopathologist [17]. Berman et al. identified a concordance rate of 80% with a variety of dermatologic entities in a retrospective analysis involving the same dermatopathologist 1 year later. The concordance rate improved to 84% with the addition of a clinical history and to 99% with the application of traditional microscopy [1]. Ferrara et al. found a diagnostic accuracy of 100% in a combined dermoscopic–pathological approach to the telediagnosis of 12 melanocytic skin neoplasms [7]. These studies suggest that diagnostic efficacy and accuracy in teledermatopathology may be particularly weak when examining entities that require the identification of subtle architectural arrangements or delicate cytologic features, as in inflammatory skin diseases [1, 2, 4, 6, 7, 16–19, 22].

Advantages and disadvantages of SAF teledermatology can be identified; for beginners basic informatics knowledge is required, but the application is relatively easy and fast to use. Nowadays almost all modern microscopes are equipped with a photographic camera adaptor, reducing the cost of SAF teledermatopathology. A photographic digital camera and a personal computer with Internet connection are the minimum equipments required that can be associated to a specific image software.

A very important issue of SAF teledermatopathology concerns image selection and quality. Image quality depends on two basic points: image acquisition and photo-editing. The current available digital photo-cameras can acquire high-resolution images; even at high magnifications these systems produce excellent images. At low magnification (scanning, 20×), the image quality is not satisfactory and cannot be compared to conventional microscopy. A special consideration should be made about the image distribution, because some microscopes do not distribute the light on the slide in a uniform manner, causing an overexposure in the center and black shadow at the periphery of the image. This particular problem can be overcome by acquiring multiple images of different fields at a higher magnification (i.e., 100×), which in a second time can be assembled together, creating just one image using special software (i.e., Panorama). None of the aforementioned studies attributed their errors to image quality [1, 2, 4, 6, 7, 16–19, 22]. The process of photo-edition using specific image software can enhance the image quality but requires special skills and experience to obtain good results. For example, in these software applications, the user can find a specific tool for automatic correction of colors and contrast, which is usually not enough for histopathologic images requiring a more sophisticated photo-editing process (see Fig. 13.1a–c).

Image selection is the second major issue concerning SAF teledermatopathology. To achieve a correct histopathologic diagnosis, the image selection becomes critical, even for expert observers. A referring pathologist who correctly establishes a reliable differential diagnosis will be able to identify which morphologic elements of the case need an expert interpretation. On the contrary, a referring pathologist who does not formulate a plausible differential diagnosis

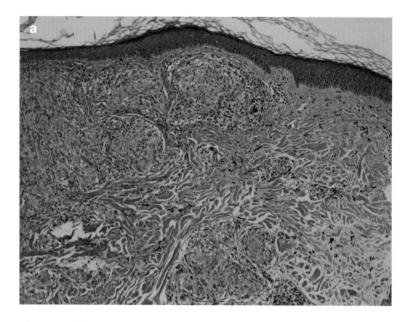

Fig. 13.1. (**a**) Sarcoidosis. Original image acquired with a conventional microscope (Eclipse E1000M, Nikon, Tokyo, Japan) and with a normal digital camera (Nikon DM 100). Image not photo-edited. The image is a little bit dark and pale (original magnification: ×100). (**b**) Same image as (**a**). Photo-edited with Photoshop, performing the automatic correction of levels, colors, and contrast. The epidermis is *dark gray* (originally in the hematoxylin & eosin slide it is blue-violet), the dermis is *pale red*, and the granulomas are *gray* (originally in the hematoxylin & eosin slide these are light blue) (original magnification: ×100). (**c**) Same image as (**a**) and (**b**). Photo-edited with Photoshop, performing only a manual correction of levels and contrast. The epidermis is *violet*, the dermis is *red*, and the granulomas are *blue-gray* (original magnification: ×100)

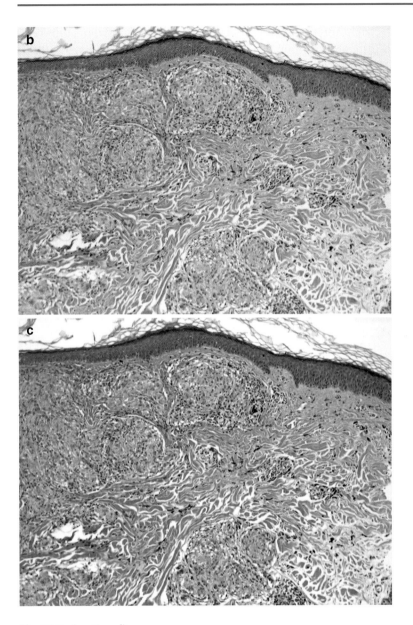

Fig. 13.1. (continued)

will most probably not select the appropriate images for consultation, thus deviating the correct interpretation of the expert. Indeed, the selection issue becomes crucial when particular features are clues for diagnoses. The search of specific features initiates at the low-power optical examination of the entire lesion and finishes with a picture at high-power magnification. Misdiagnosis caused by the lack of submission of correct images is termed "field selection error." This type of error was reported in three of the aforementioned studies and not only in skin pathology but also in many other organ systems [2].

Even highly expert dermatopathologists encounter serious difficulties in performing diagnoses in difficult cases; this premise can be applied also for SAF teledermatopathology. So, the users of this system of expert consultation should be conscious of the individual limitations regarding particular cases. In some cases, the result will just only refute or confirm the baseline proposal. In particular, if a diagnosis should be done by exclusion of other diseases, SAF teledermatopathology will require more images, a profound clinical background, and an accurate follow-up of the patient to contribute to the final definitive diagnoses.

13.3
Real-Time (Dynamic) Teledermatopathology

This approach attempt to reproduce a dynamic screening by live, full-motion, remotely controlled video microscopy. Real-time teledermatopathology is more appealing to most pathologists because it closely resembles the established technique of pathologic examination. However, it requires a high quality of communication to transmit video images. Economical limitations are referred to software and hardware applications and to the availability of high fidelity telecommunication [2].

Morgan et al. tested the efficiency and reproducibility of dynamic teledermatopathology comparing the diagnoses on 100 specimens (25 melanocytic lesions, 50 nonmelanoma skin cancers, and 25 inflammatory dermatoses), rendered by two independent, board-certified dermatopathologists, using a double-headed microscope and teledermatopathology from two remote sites (approximately 64 km apart) [16]. The two-headed microscopes used for both arms of this study were the Olympus model BX-40 (Olympus, Tokyo, Japan). Each telepathology microscope was fitted with a Sharp XG-A1 color camera (Sharp, Tokyo, Japan). The image was compressed and transmitted by a V-TEL LC 5000 video codec (Rockledge, FL, USA), using Apps View Smart Video conferencing software (Windows 95-based v1.00.06; Microsoft Corporation, Redmond, WA, USA). The image was sent through T1 line at 768 kB/s using a multiband transmitter (V-TEL Enterprise series, Model LX-2). The transmitted image was received through a reciprocal personal computer running the identical V-TEC code and software. It was then processed and sent at a resolution of 640 × 480 active lines through an RG-59 cable to a Sony 27-inch Trinitron monitor (Tokyo, Japan). A separate voice-transmittal speakphone line was present at each facility. The agreement for teledermatopathology ($\kappa = 0.76$) was good, whereas the agreement with conventional two-headed microscopy was better ($\kappa = 0.93$). With real-time teledermatopathology, the pathologists were able to generate remote telediagnoses in less than 1 min per slide for random, unselected cases. Conclusions of this study were that although diagnostic accuracy and time taken per case were acceptable with video-assisted diagnosis, conventional microscope had significantly higher accuracy and shorter time per diagnosis. However, in clinical practice, dynamic teledermatopathology does not appear to present a serious time limitation, given the proper equipment and expertise of the operators [16].

13.4
Virtual Microscope Teledermatopathology

In the last several years, hybrid systems that combine limited robotic capabilities with high-resolution images (VSS) have been introduced in telepathology. The new VSSs are digital facsimiles of the visual content of glass microscope slides acquired at high magnification. In this technique, a conventionally prepared glass slide is placed on a microscope with a motorized stage and automatic focus facility. The slide is scanned using a 20× or 40× objective lens, and these images are integrated to produce a single large image file [3,21]. This file can then be viewed on any computer at any location with a virtual microscope interface, where a user can press any keys to change magnification from an overall low power to the resolution at which it was scanned (Fig. 13.2a–d) [3,21]. An important concern of this technique relies on the positioning of the image, where an orthogonal disposition of the tissue in the slide border becomes mandatory to avoid an image oriented upside-down. In this way, the major limitations concerning SAF teledermatopathology imposed by capturing small preselected areas and subjective sampling can be overcome. This technique holds a huge potential of development; with the introduction of an automatic slide feeder, the user would be able to produce slides in digital format that can be used in daily routine diagnostic work. The digital format slide created by this system can be used in any location, for example, on a computer in a multidisciplinary team meeting room, saving time-consuming searching and sorting of glass slides. The application of this technique is still limited by economical concerns (cost of equipment) and by slow-transmitting connections related to the scarcity of broadband lines [9,16,21]. Some web-based versions of virtual microscope

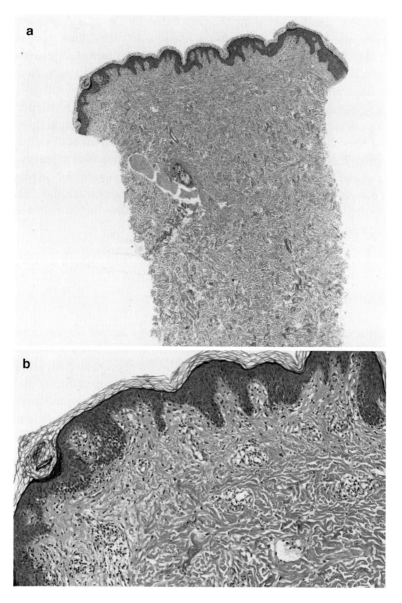

Fig. 13.2. Images from a virtual microscope (Aperio, Aperio Technologies, Inc., Vista, CA, USA). Starting from the single image file (which is an SVS file, 49 MB in size), a user can press any keys to change magnification from an overall low power (**a**) to medium power (**b**, **c**), till to the resolution at which it was scanned (×40) (**d**). Notice that there is no decrease in image resolution with the increasing simulated magnification (the specimen was scanned using a real ×40 objective lens). An important concern of this technique relies on the positioning of the image, where an orthogonal disposition of the tissue in the slide border becomes mandatory to avoid an image oriented upside-down

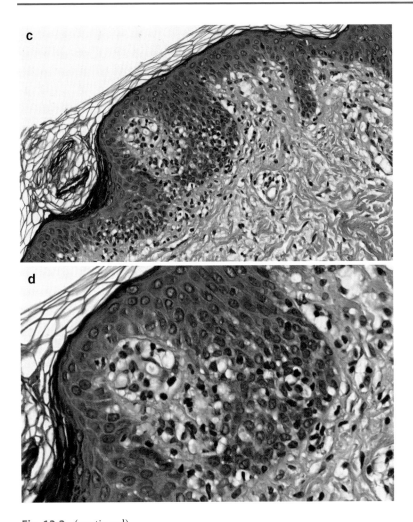

Fig. 13.2. (continued)

(i.e., http://telederm.org/research/dermatopath/default.asp, http://www.web-microscope.net/, http://alf3.urz.unibas.ch/vmic/list.cfm, and http://interpath1.uio.no/telemedisin/WebInterPath/interpathindex.htm) [5, 21, 15] have been developed, which reduce transmission problems by transmitting only those fields that are immediately required by the viewer. Images stored on a VS server are accessible to multiple users simultaneously. The images are still of diagnostic quality, and this system could be used for many purposes, from routine work to education for medical students or self-assessment courses [8, 23].

Although this technology has existed for more than a decade, this process has been commercially available only since 1998 [21]. Helin et al. evaluated the validity of a web-based virtual microscopy for Gleason grading in prostatic carcinoma and found an intraobserver agreement with identical Gleason score in 48 of 62 cases ($\kappa = 0.73$) and a difference of only 1 point in the remaining 14 cases [9]. Dee et al. evaluated the teaching modality of VSS and showed that VSS enhanced student's ability to grasp morphological features better than the traditional photo-micrographs [5]. Glatz-Krieger et al. applied the VSS technology for teaching purpose with a new type of web-based VSS [8]. Ultrarapid VS processors have recently been developed, and Weinstein et al. found a κ of 0.96 among the diagnosis on the VSs obtained with ultrarapid VSS and the conventional light microscopy studying 30 breast surgical pathology cases [24]. Moreover, VSSs are already being used for pathology diagnostic services applications [12, 13].

Only few experiences have been reported concerning the use of VSS in teledermatopathology. Leinweber et al. focused on the technical requirements for achievement of a correct diagnosis on digital histopathologic images [11]. A collection of 560 melanocytic lesions was selected from the files of the Department of Dermatology, Medical University of Graz, Austria. From each lesion, one histologic slide was completely digitally scanned with a robotic microscope. Digital scanning was performed with an Axioplan II imaging microscope (Zeiss, Oberkochen, Germany) using a motorized scanning table and automatic focus facilities, which were navigated by the KS4003.0 image analysis system (ZeissVision, Halbergmoos, Germany), a second-generation VS processor of "Class 4A" (according to the classification of Weinstein et al. on telepathology systems) [10, 23]. The image analysis software used also allowed, apart from scanning, focusing, recording, and storing, a reproduction of images in different magnifications and image details. Image recording was performed with a Sony CCD video camera (Sony, Tokyo, Japan). For each specimen, a meander, comprising the whole lesion, was defined by choosing two opposite corners. Subsequently, the meander was gradually scanned with a 40× objective, resulting in a magnification of 0.33 mm per pixel. All captured single-picture fields were merged by the image analysis system to the full picture and subsequently saved together with a white reference as compressed JPEG files on a central server. Digital pictures were reviewed by four dermatopathologists using a presentation program, which recorded the number of image calls, applied magnifications, overall time needed, and amount of transmitted bits during the digital sign-out. One month later, the four microscopists had to review the corresponding slides and render a direct diagnosis on each case. Telepathologic diagnoses corresponded with the original diagnoses in a range from 90.4% to 96.4% of cases (κ, 0.80–0.93; P, 0.001). The median time needed for achievement of a diagnosis was 22 s and was significantly higher for melanomas compared with nevi. The median transmission effort for each diagnosis was 510 kB after JPEG compression using an ISDN line with a transmission capacity of 64 kb/s; this correlates to a transmission time of about 1 min. The authors concluded that correct reporting on digital histopathologic images is possible with only a little time exposure. For an adequately fast transmission, ISDN lines are sufficient after JPEG compression [15].

Massone et al. performed the first specific study in teledermatopathology using VSS focusing only on inflammatory skin diseases [15]. Twelve teleconsultants from six different countries were asked to report 46 cases recruited from the routine collection of the Research Unit for Dermatopathology, Medical University of Graz, Austria. Specimens were selected on the basis of their quality and their diagnosis in order to cover a broad spectrum of cutaneous inflammatory diseases. The conventional diagnosis was based on the histopathologic evaluation together with the given clinical data, using a conventional light microscope. The gold standard diagnosis was proved by two experienced dermatopathologists, based on histopathologic findings with given clinical data and, in addition, clinical follow-up visits for performing a clinicopathologic correlation, including relevant laboratory data. Digitalized images of each slide were obtained by scanning at 20× optical magnification with a Nikon Eclipse E-400 two-headed microscope connected to the Morphoscan™ robotic platform, connected with a high-resolution digital camera (Hamamatsu C4749-95), a second-generation VS processor of "Class 4A" (according to the classification of Weinsten et al. on telepathology systems), which allows performing a high-resolution automatic acquisition of tissue sections [3, 23]. The image software integrated and created digital high-resolution images of the whole skin specimen. Fifty-five images (46 hematoxylin & eosin specimens and nine periodic acid-Schiff (PAS) stains) were first acquired in TIFF format and then compressed in JPEG format by Imstar software with a compression ratio of 80% (average size of JPEG files). Final image size ranged from 3,769 × 3,308 to 6,907 × 14,553 pixels in RGB color mode (24 bits). Images were then saved on a computer with a Pentium IV CPU 1.8 GHz and 516 MB RAM. No photo-editing has been performed on the images. As a second step, the digital images as originally acquired with the Imstar system were uploaded on the server of a specific web application suited for telepathology (http://telederm.org/research/dermatopath/default.asp). This server is login and password protected and only available to the participants of this study [14,20]. The web application integrates an image viewer software (WebScope©) and works in a manner that closely resembles a light microscope. The interface included an overall low-power view of the specimen on the left side of the screen, which provided an aid to navigation on the image. Different zoom modalities allowed various magnifications of the specimens up to the resolution at which they have been scanned, without decrease in image definition. Sample images of this study are available on the World Wide Web at http:// telederm.org/research/dermatopath/. The images may be navigated using the image viewer software WebScope©.

For each case, clinical data and histopathologic images were available directly on the web application. Clinical history, location, and clinical differential diagnosis were given exactly as they were reported on the original request slip. Complete clinical data were, in this way, available only for 36 cases. Each participant to this study was given a unique login and password and reviewed independently all VSs simply by connecting directly on the web application. No specific software download was required. Even if it is difficult to compare results of this study with those of the literature, the percentage of correct telediagnoses (73%) is the lowest ever reported [1, 2, 4, 6, 7, 16–19, 22]. Theoretically, the teleconsultants of this study were in the most appropriate conditions to make the correct telediagnoses, having at their disposal a virtual microscope with high-resolution images and complete clinical data available for most of the cases. It seems that results have not been influenced by lack of knowledge in dermatopathology, all the teleconsultants being either experienced pathologists or dermatopathologists. A complete concordance of telediagnosis with both conventional and gold-standard diagnosis was achieved in nine cases. The comparison of the telediagnoses with the conventional diagnoses may better reflect the real routine setting. Even if there was no global numerical difference among the average of correct telediagnoses with the gold-standard diagnoses and with the conventional diagnoses (73% vs. 74%), in some cases the conventional diagnosis was tricky and initially equivocal. Final diagnoses were achieved only after an accurate and complete clinicopathologic correlation, including additional laboratory data. This fact might explain partially the high number of incorrect diagnoses in some cases. Possible other explanations are the intrinsic difficulties of cutaneous inflammatory pathology. In fact, subtle changes of the arrangement of the inflammatory infiltrate or a slight difference in the architectural pattern may create a degree of variability in the morphologic appearance of a given inflammatory skin disease, making the histopathologic diagnosis extremely difficult. Moreover, it seems likely that the lack of complete clinical data in 10 cases negatively influenced the percentage of correct telediagnoses. There was a notable discrepancy between the average of concordance of telediagnosis without and with complete clinical data with gold-standard diagnoses (65% vs. 75%, respectively) and the average of concordance of telediagnosis without and with complete clinical data with conventional diagnoses (66% vs. 76%, respectively). Another limitation of this study might have been the reality that the teleconsultants were not yet very familiar with the use of a virtual microscope. It is possible that with VSS the identification of diagnostic clues leading to the correct diagnosis is more difficult compared to the use of a conventional microscope. According to the teleconsultants, it seems likely that there have not been any hardware/software limitations in this study. Three of the teleconsultants signaled problems in the image downloading being, in some cases, very slow. This problem seems to be related rather by the Internet connection than by the web application used. In fact, the images in this study were saved on the server of the web application; the WebScope© software integrated in the web application elaborated the images directly on the server of telederm. org/research, and only the part of the images concerning the fields and magnifications selected by the teleconsultants were downloaded. In this way, all images downloaded had about the same size for the teleconsultants. The sizes of the images to download varied from about 150–250 kB independently of the original size of the image stored on the server (this was up to 60 MB JPEG files). The downloading time for the images in the case of a dial-up connection of 56 kb/s was about 20–35 s and in the case of a connection of 1 Mb/s it was about 7–12 s.

It must be underlined that even if all cases of this study have been studied without signaling technical defects and even if the global judgment on the image quality according to the teleconsultants was positive, the image quality still might have represented a limitation. Images acquired with VSS, in general, are far from being perfect and these are not as good as what one would see looking down the microscope. The main issue of acquiring images with a VSS concerns the focusing system. In fact, VSS devices have usually excellent optics, but to perform the autofocusing, the camera has to sample the image and the sampling process is virtually always far "coarser" than the sampling by the human eye. Moreover, the image is compressed. Weinstein et al. studied the quality of the 30 images of breast surgical pathology cases acquired with an the ultrarapid VS processor (DMetrix DX-40); four case readers had to score the image quality using a Linker-type rating scale, and results showed that 56.6% of the image ratings were 4 (excellent), 39.2% of the image ratings were 3 (good), 4.2% of the image ratings were 2 (fair), and none of the image ratings were 1 (poor). Image quality ratings were highest for cases reported as benign (mean = 3.53) and malignant (mean = 3.5), followed closely by cases reported as equivocal diagnoses (mean = 3.33) [24]. These data show that image quality still represent a not completely resolved issue in VSS. Massone et al. concluded that despite its usability, VSS are not completely feasible for teledermatopathology of inflammatory skin diseases. In fact, only three out of four cases of inflammatory skin diseases were correctly diagnosed. Moreover, the performance seems to have been influenced by the availability of complete clinical data and by the intrinsic difficulty of the pathology of inflammatory skin diseases [15].

13.5
Conclusions

Even if SAF teledermatopathology is still the most frequently used and less expensive approach to teledermatopathology, VSS represents the future in this discipline. As technology continues to look forward, problems reported in previous literature reports are becoming less frequent. Actually the economical investment for VSS or real-time teledermatopathology equipments may be beyond the reach of most dermatopathology practices, but not faraway from tomorrow when high-resolution devices will become accessible for most of us [16]. The recent pilot studies suggest that the use of remote expert consultants in diagnostic dermatopathology can be integrated into the daily routine [15,24]. This technology enables rapid and reproducible diagnoses, even though problems are basically found in the intrinsic difficulty of interpreting dermatopathology of inflammatory and neoplastic skin diseases, particularly in the context of lack of complete clinical data. Further development of the VSS, continuous research on the new VS processor, and further training in the virtual microscope will help to improve the diagnostic performance of teleconsultants.

13.6
Summary

- Teledermatopathology can be performed with real-time (dynamic) transmission of images or the store-and-forward (SAF; static) option.
- The real-time method provides remote consultation via a robotic microscope, which can be controlled by the consulting pathologist. It requires a high quality of communication to transmit video images. Economical limitations are referred to software and hardware applications and to the availability of high fidelity telecommunication.
- With SAF system, each image is captured and transmitted as a single file. The fields to be examined are selected by the referring pathologist and then transmitted by e-mail or FTP connection or using specific web applications. This method is relatively cheap, easy, and fast to use but the image selection is a major issue.
- Recently, VSSs have been introduced. With these systems the whole slide can be digitized at high resolution, which allows the user to view any part of the specimen at any magnification. In this way, the limitations imposed by capturing small preselected areas can be overcome. Moreover, the acquired images can be stored on a VS server that makes them available on the web, and an integrated VS client enables the users to browse the VS.

- The feasibility of both SAF and real-time teledermatopathology has been proven in few studies, mainly on nonmelanoma skin cancer or on melanocytic lesions, suggesting that diagnostic efficacy and accuracy in teledermatopathology may be particularly weak when examining entities that require the identification of subtle architectural arrangements or delicate cytologic features, as in inflammatory skin diseases.
- Recent studies investigated the feasibility of VSS in teledermatopathology both on melanocytic lesions and on inflammatory skin diseases and confirmed the intrinsic difficulties of dermatopathology. However, this technique holds a huge potential of development and represents the future in this discipline.

References

1. Berman B, Elgart GW, Burdick AE (1997) Dermatopathology via a still-image telemedicine system: diagnostic concordance with direct microscopy. Telemed J 3:27–32
2. Black-Schaffer S, Flotte TJ (2001) Teledermatopathology. Adv Dermatol 17:325–338
3. Cross SS, Dennis T, Start RD (2002) Telepathology: current status and future prospects in diagnostic histopathology. Histopathology 41:91–109
4. Dawson PJ, Johnson JG, Edgemon LJ, et al. (2000) Outpatient frozen sections by telepathology in a Veterans Administration medical center. Hum Pathol 31:786–788
5. Dee FR, Lehman JM, Consoer D, et al. (2003) Implementation of virtual microscope slides in the annual pathobiology of cancer workshop laboratory. Hum Pathol 34:430–436
6. Della Mea V, Puglisi F, Forti S, et al. (1997) Expert pathology consultation through the Internet: melanoma vs benign melanocytic tumours. J Telemed Telecare 3(Suppl 1):17–79
7. Ferrara G, Argenziano G, Cerroni L, et al. (2004) A pilot study of a combined dermoscopic-pathological approach to the telediagnosis of melanocytic skin neoplasms. J Telemed Telecare 10:34–38
8. Glatz-Krieger K, Glatz D, Mihatsch MJ (2003) Virtual slides: high-quality demand, physical limitations, and affordability. Hum Pathol 34:968–974
9. Helin H, Lundin M, Lundin J, et al. (2005) Web-based virtual microscopy in teaching and standardizing Gleason grading. Hum Pathol 36:381–386
10. KS400 Imaging System Release 3.0 (1997) CarlZeissVision, Munich
11. Leinweber B, Massone C, Kodama K, et al. (2006) Teledermatopathology: a controlled study about diagnostic validity and technical requirements for digital transmission. Am J Dermatopathol 28:413–416
12. Leong AS, Leong FJ (2005) Strategies for laboratory cost containment and for pathologist shortage: centralised pathology laboratories with microwave-stimulated histoprocessing and telepathology. Pathology 37:5–9
13. Lundin M, Lundin J, Helin H, Isola J (2004) A digital atlas of breast histopathology: an application of web based virtual microscopy. J Clin Pathol 57:1288–1291
14. Massone C, Soyer HP, Hofmann-Wellenhof R, et al. (2006) Two years' experience with Web-based teleconsulting in dermatology. J Telemed Telecare 12:83–87
15. Massone C, Soyer HP, Lozzi GP, et al. (2007) Feasibility and diagnostic agreement in teledermatopathology using a virtual slide system. Hum Pathol 38:546–554

16. Morgan MB, Tannenbaum M, Smoller BR (2003) Telepathology in the diagnosis of routine dermatopathologic entities. Arch Dermatol 139:637–640
17. Okada DH, Binder SW, Felten CL, et al. (1999) "Virtual microscopy" and the internet as telepathology consultation tools: diagnostic accuracy in evaluating melanocytic skin lesions. Am J Dermatopathol 21:525–531
18. Pak HS (2002) Teledermatology and teledermatopathology. Semin Cutan Med Surg 21:179–189
19. Piccolo D, Soyer HP, Burgdorf W, et al. (2002) Concordance between telepathologic diagnosis and conventional histopathologic diagnosis: a multiobserver store-and-forward study on 20 skin specimens. Arch Dermatol 138:53–58
20. Soyer HP, Hofmann-Wellenhof R, Massone C, et al. (2005) telederm.org: freely available online consultations in dermatology. PLoS Med 2:e87
21. Weinstein RS (2005) Innovations in medical imaging and virtual microscopy. Hum Pathol 36:317–319
22. Weinstein LJ, Epstein JI, Edlow D, Westra WH (1997) Static image analysis of skin specimens: the application of telepathology to frozen section evaluation. Hum Pathol 28:30–35
23. Weinstein RS, Descour MR, Liang C, et al. (2001) Telepathology overview: from concept to implementation. Hum Pathol 32:1283–1299
24. Weinstein RS, Descour MR, Liang C, et al. (2004) An array microscope for ultrarapid virtual slide processing and telepathology. Design, fabrication, and validation study. Hum Pathol 35:1303–1314

Ultrastructural Telepathology: Remote EM Diagnostic via Internet

Josef A. Schroeder

14.1
Introduction

Pathology, a diagnostic medical discipline, is associated in the mind of most people with performing autopsies on human bodies to find out the reason for death. This traditional understanding of anatomical pathology is conveyed in numerous works of narrative and fine art, for example, the famous canvas "The Anatomy Lesson of Dr. Tulp" painted in 1632 by Rembrandt van Rijn [77] or the impressive contemporary "Body Worlds" exhibitions of Gunther von Hagens [39], which is attracting considerable interest and controversy.

However, in fact, modern pathologists are mainly occupied with the light microscopy examination of cells (e.g., smears of exfoliated cells and fine-needle aspirations) and tissue or organ excisions (surgical pathology) from living patients with a disease. The patient's clinician needs a cytology or tissue-based diagnosis describing the nature of the lesion and an interpretation of the data providing advice for an individual therapeutic strategy. The precedent for the shift in the pathological focus to the "living patient" was Virchow's cellular theory, dating from 1858: this inaugurated the change from the ancient Hippocratic body fluid "humoral pathology" to contemporary "cellular pathology" and provided explanations of several observations – then considered strange – such as inflammation, infection, or cancer at the light microscopic level ("think microscopic") [98]. It has taken more than a century to develop the microscopy and laboratory technology (tissue fixation, cutting, and staining) and the interpretation of tissue and cellular structure in terms of diagnostic features.

Today, tissue-based diagnosis is the "gold standard" for all subsequent medical procedures, especially surgery or drug treatment, and has a pronounced specificity and sensitivity in terms of clinical significance. Recent achievements in molecular biology and genetics using the nucleic acid amplification technique (polymerase chain reaction, PCR), combined with microscopic investigation such as in situ hybridization (FISH) and tissue microarray (TMA) processing

[22, 27, 51, 78, 101], provide a more detailed and "time-related" insight into the pathways of disease: we can now discern classic and prognosis-, risk-, and treatment-associated diagnoses. The complexities of these new techniques in concert with modern information technology (IT) have had a great impact on current pathology practice and may well lead to a paradigm shift for the discipline, partly but not only due to this new methodology [1, 12, 65, 76, 79].

In contrast to the extended responsibilities of pathologists as a result of the new genomics, proteomics, and metabolomics, the histopathologic diagnosis is still primarily based on the light microscopic examination of a classical hematoxylin and eosin (H&E)-stained, 4–7 µm thin tissue section mounted on a glass slide. This tissue visualization technique, perfected over the years, "fixes" the spatial arrangement of a living biological system as tissue or organ morphology (architecture), which is the phenotypic expression of the genetic information coded in the DNA in the cell nucleus (= genotype). Using the H&E and special staining procedures, one can analyze the important biological structures in normal healthy tissues and their disturbance under conditions of abnormality (disease). Until now, particularly abnormal tissue growth could not be treated without knowledge of the tumor morphology [101]. If the analyzed features are smaller than the resolution limit of the light microscope (200 nm), the 1,000 times higher resolving power of electron microscope (EM) technology (0.2 nm) can provide ultrastructural data at the subcellular level to facilitate a diagnosis that might be uncertain by light microscopy [20, 28]. To assess the functional status of a lesion or abnormal growth, other techniques, for example, immunohistochemistry [101], can visualize the expression of specific "marker" macromolecules, providing a simple "yes–no" presence or absence of a characteristic molecule, for example, breast cancer receptor protein or antigen.

In both light and electron microscopic images, the information content is separated intuitively by the observer into two diagnostically relevant domains: an object-associated information and a nonobject-related part (=background). The objects usually display "abnormal" features (cancer or inflammatory cells, inclusions, and infectious agents), which are not present in the analyzed tissue under normal (healthy) conditions. Once detected, the specific object features allow, for example, a biological classification (cell type, bacterium, or virus) or identification of structural and functional units (glands, vessels, mitochondria, or filaments). In many samples, also the background and its context or texture can contain valuable information (grey values, basic pattern, and relations to the object) to help reach the right diagnosis. Because each pathologist has his/her own algorithm for the image analysis and interpretation, in difficult cases it can happen that different pathologists can give different diagnostic statements (interpretations) on the same specimen [49, 101].

This problem of interobserver variability can be solved by a group discussion of the case using a multiheaded microscope, as shown in Fig. 14.1, or a consensus

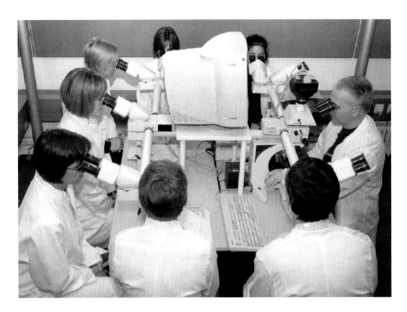

Fig. 14.1. Traditional local and simultaneous image sharing at a multiheaded light microscope during the intradepartmental daily case discussion. Every observer can see exactly the same tissue image area at the magnification chosen by the case-referring pathologist and make comments on the rendered diagnosis. (Courtesy of Pathology Department University Hospital/Regensburg)

report of a panel board discussion (mandatory in several countries, e.g., hematological tumors), or by consultation of a recognized expert or reference center for this special case/disease. The simple and traditional way of requesting a "second opinion" was to send the glass slides with the tissue sections (optionally also the paraffin blocks for preparing additional sections if necessary) by "snail" mail and wait for the expert's statement. The answer was usually available after some days or weeks.

Another time delay aspect is related to "frozen-section diagnosis service," which is usually requested to guide the surgeon intraoperatively [75]. Particularly in smaller hospitals, which cannot afford to employ a pathologist and which may be located in remote or impassable country areas, the excised tissue or tumor samples are transported by courier to an urban "hub" pathology center for cryostat sectioning and "crude" diagnosis (time can be crucial, because the patient is still under anesthesia). The instantaneous advice of the pathologist (e.g., in assessing excision margins for a tumor) is essential for the course and extension of the surgical treatment. Clearly, therefore, some diagnoses are very urgent or of great impact for the patient's treatment, and a great deal of effort has gone into improving these procedures, which include digital technology.

14.2
The Digital Era

The real breakthrough in rapid sharing of medical information independent of place, distance, and time has been made possible by fast-paced computer, Internet, and telecommunication technologies. The digital revolution has given rise to new tools and techniques in different disciplines of science; mobile messaging and video-streaming has become a daily experience for ordinary people, but more exciting – during the last decade the Internet has enabled people to have firsthand worldwide access to information and, for example, appreciate remote operation of complex space mission devices such as the "Sojourner" (1996, Pathfinder Mars Mission) or the "Spirit" rover roboter (2004) performing microscopic and spectroscopic analyses of rocks on Mars [67]. Much of this new knowledge has been assimilated into different telemedicine applications (tele-diagnosis, teletherapy, telecare, tele-education, teleresearch, telemeasurement, and administration) [10,11,13,16,33,38,44,56,73,80,88,100] and has been implemented by morphologists to study microscopic samples. "Telepresence microscopy" [113] is a term coined in 1998 and includes the remote operation of microscopes using telecommunication links or the Internet, applied to pathology in the fields of light and electron microscopy (EM).

14.3
From Remote to Virtual Light Microscopy

Interestingly, the first concept of performing a diagnosis at a distance was born in the very early days of radio broadcast development and is illustrated in the "Radio News" of 1924 [107]. However, for regular distant expert consultations, live black-and-white images of skin and blood diseases were first transmitted from Logan Airport to the Massachusetts General Hospital in Boston using a broadband telecommunication system in 1968. In 1985, Dr. R.S. Weinstein demonstrated the high diagnostic accuracy of video microscopy, while in 1986 he installed the first "robotic" light microscope for transmission of real-time images from El Paso/Texas to Washington DC via an SBS-3Comsat satellite [102,103]. In 1989 in Europe, in the rural areas of Norway, two provincial hospitals, without their own pathologist, installed a robotic pathology diagnostic system (a telephone/video combination) and were linked to the University of Tromsö Pathology Department, providing them with intraoperative frozen-section support. In February 1990, the first remote expert consultation was performed in Germany, between Darmstadt, Hannover, and Mainz [46,102]. The rapid progress in digital sensor technique and digital image processing and increasing bandwidth of telecommunication links attracted increasing numbers of researchers and institutions to use this new technology for collaboration in science and health; the collected experience was shared at the first European Telepathology Conference in Heidelberg in 1992.

Today, one can speak of fourth-generation telepathology systems (=diagnostic pathology service at a distance, SNOMED definition), the technology having matured to the point where light microscopy telepathology has become a standard tool in a number of clinics and hospitals worldwide, and its applicability to and suitability for diagnostic routine use are well documented [46,104,105]. It includes a wide range of possible telepathology applications from remote gross (macroscopic) specimen description [55], intraoperative frozen section service [6,14,15,17,43,68,106,109], request for a second opinion [21,72,91,92,103,115], and quality assurance in screening pathology [40,47] to distance learning [2,7,46,53,73], using commercial systems. They are working in a passive (store and forward) or active (real-time) telepathology mode. The passive systems acquire and digitize images from a microscope and transmit them to a remote site for a second opinion; the recipient has no control over the image sampling, magnification, and quality and must trust the transmitting participant to have selected an adequate area of specimen. The dynamic or real-time telepathology systems give the remote expert as much control over the image selection as the sender. By remote control of the microscope, the expert can get an overview of the specimen at low magnification, select the relevant areas of interest, and choose the appropriate magnification to render a diagnosis. In this new millennium, an automated procedure has been described [19], capable of managing a robotic microscope and rapid image acquisition for the construction of a "virtual case": this consists of a "stitched-up" collection of digital images ("tiles") from a histological/cytological slide at all magnification levels together with all relevant clinical data. This "digital slide" can be viewed on a computer using a user-friendly interface ("digital microscope") and used for multiple purposes independent of time and space with respect to the observer. To reduce the time necessary for scanning the original glass slide, this trend culminated in the development of a miniaturized light microscope array (MMA), allowing ultrarapid virtual slide processing [37,49,105].

14.4
Implications for Diagnostic Electron Microscopy

These developments were not applied to the use of EM for remote diagnostic applications, and there are several reasons for this. On the one hand, this may be due to the general decline of the use of EM in recent decades due to major advances in immunohistochemistry and molecular techniques (in situ hybridization, PCR). On the other hand, in addition to applications in research, the diagnostic value of EM in surgical pathology [29,30,95] in such areas as renal, muscle, nervous system, skin, ciliary defects, storage diseases, opportunistic infections, and rapid viral diagnosis is good [20,28,31,35,70]. Diagnostic EM possesses an approximately 100 times higher resolution as light microscopy, and so it visualizes structures not recognizable by light microscopy examination. In combination with rapid microwave-assisted tissue preparation procedures [25,50,84], it can deliver specific and exact findings on the same day as sampling and make therapeutic decisions that are much easier. It is important to realize that the ultrastructural examination of neoplasms, especially addressing diagnostic difficulties by light microscopy, is a complementary approach with other techniques such as immunohistochemistry [32,42,69] and can be a very valuable adjunct to diagnostic assessment (including samples retrieved from tissues previously embedded in paraffin).

Another example is rapid viral diagnosis: in the negative-staining method, viruses are applied directly to a small grid coated with a support film and can be visualized in approximately half an hour after sample arrival (Fig. 14.2). No agent-specific

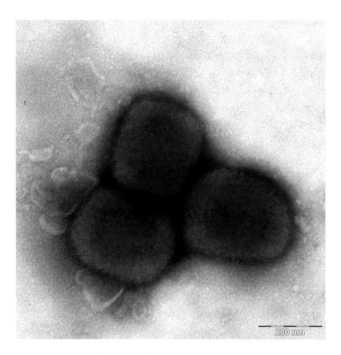

200 nm

Fig. 14.2. Digital image of poxviruses, prepared with the rapid negative-staining method (2% PTA) and visualized half an hour later in the EM. This mouse ectromelia virus belongs to the poxvirus family, and its morphology and size are identical to the small-pox particles, which have a bioterrorism potential. Original magnification ×40,000. (Sample courtesy of N. Bannert, Robert-Koch-Institute/Berlin)

solutions or antigens are necessary, and, owing to the "open view" of the experienced observer, multiple or totally unexpected infectious agents can be detected [58,70].

Second, owing to a reduction in the demand for diagnostic EM examinations in the last two decades and the need to limit laboratory running costs, the microscopy equipment is often technically not up to date in many laboratories. An analog-operated EM with a traditional photographic plate camera is not suitable for remote control and effective networking. This situation is slowly changing, because now (often for economic reasons) centralized EM units, equipped with modern digitally controlled EMs and digital image acquisition, are being established in life-science centers and clinics. Another point is the lack of automation and rationalization of the sample preparation and embedding methods. The implementation of micro-processor-controlled tissue processors and use of microwave-assisted procedures are considerably reducing sample turnaround times (from 3–4 days to a matter of hours); in short, "same day" diagnoses are becoming a clinical reality [84].

Third, the virtual slide concept [37,49] – so promising for light microscopy – can probably not be applied for virtual EM. The intrinsic problem is the grid (equivalent to the glass slide) carrying the tissue section, with its bars partitioning the section into translucent and obscured parts, and this creates currently a number of problems in correct image acquisition with a digital camera: alignment of multiple image "tiles" into one large picture ("virtual slide") is very problematic. Another challenge is the different modes in which samples are examined in light microscopy and EM, the latter having an inherent and considerable magnification range. This means that, compared with virtual light microscopy, different technical solutions may be needed for EM.

14.5
The Need for Ultrastructural Telepathology

With the realization among many surgical pathologists that immunohisto-chemistry and the current rapidly evolving molecular procedures are not capable of resolving all diagnostic problems, there has been a resurgence of interest in transmission EM as an ancillary diagnostic tool [29,32,61]. In our opinion, the value and usefulness of ultrastructural examinations could be increased greatly by establishing a worldwide consultation network of experts or "national centers of excellence" to assist in obtaining and interpreting ultrastructural data of complex cases in real time. What is almost a consultation routine for light microscopy histopathologists (in specialized telediagnosis centers such as AFIP [108]; UICC, Berlin [21]; iPATH, Basel [8]; and WWM, Japan [66]) would be equally useful for ultrastructural pathology. The two main benefits would be time savings in "live" examination of the original specimen by remote experts and avoiding difficulties inherent in the interpretation of either photographic prints ("snail posting") or a still image collection (e-mail attachments), possibly captured from inadequate areas of the tissue in question. A significant advantage specifically of worldwide consultation networks for ultrastructural telepathology would be that expensive instrumentation would become available for remote experts or users [93]. This may be extremely useful in case of an unknown or epidemic viral outbreak (such as SARS, avian flu, and norovirus) as well as in potential bioterror scenarios [36,41,57,62,63].

14.6
Remote Electron Microscopy

The ability to examine original samples live can be realized by modern automated and digitally controlled EMs using telepresence microscopy and collaborative techniques. In materials science, several research groups around the world are already demonstrating the benefits of remote collaboration and consultation [99,111,114]. In 2000, the remote observation of thick biological samples across the Pacific was reported using the world's unique 3MV EM (Hitachi H-3000) at Osaka University [93]. The first remote examination of pathological tissue and virus samples was demonstrated live at the G7SP4 conference (Global Health Care Applications Project, Sub-Project 4) in Regensburg, in November 1998, in collaboration with the Oak Ridge National Laboratory (ORNL) TE, USA, and Edgar Voelkl and Larry Allard [81,82]. For the transatlantic sessions, the material science-oriented Hitachi HF-2000 TEM in Oak Ridge was operated remotely via the Internet using the commercial collaborative software TimbuktuPro® (http://www.Netopia.com). This software effectively mirrors the remote computer, in this case a Macintosh running the DigitalMicrograph program at ORNL, to a Windows computer at the University of Regensburg, operated by the author, J. Schroeder. A technically updated and completely remote-operable system was recently reported by the L. Allard group at the MSA 2007 conference for functional remote microscopy via the Atlantic ("Global Lab," Imperial College London, UK) [71].

14.7
The Ultrastructural Telepathology Setup

A different setup, designed in a server–client architecture and based on the LEO912AB transmission EM located at our Central EM-Lab at the University Hospital Regensburg, was introduced on 4–6 May 2000, at the Society for Cutaneous Ultrastructure Research (SCUR) Meeting in Bochum, Germany [97]. This digitally controlled EFTEM (LEO/Zeiss, Oberkochen, Germany) provides an in-column integrated energy filter, operates at 80–120 kV and is an optimal instrument for biological and diagnostic sample examination. At this time, it was equipped with a bottom-mounted 1,024 × 1,024 pixel CCD slow-scan camera (TRS˙/Moorenweis, Germany) for image acquisition. The system was controlled by a Windows NT server and acquired the images from the camera by a frame grabber. The commercial software "analySIS˙" (EsiVision˙ Ver. 3.1, SIS/Muenster) was expanded with a dedicated TelePresence server module that controlled the microscope and handled the communication with the remote computer. At the "client site" in Bochum, a laptop equipped with an ISDN-PCMCIA card provided direct access to the Internet (a client "analy-SIS˙" software was installed on the laptop computer). A video beamer with a resolution of 1,024 × 768 pixels displayed the remote examination of a (routinely prepared) skin biopsy section from a CADASIL patient to the audience (CADASIL is a central nervous system disease with ischemic stroke; the definitive diagnosis is rendered by EM evidence of specific, very small deposits in the wall of skin vessels) (Fig. 14.3). The meeting participants could not only

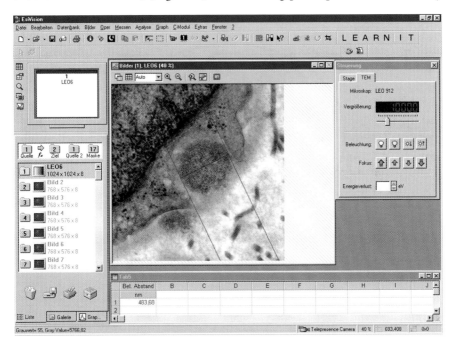

Fig. 14.3. Historical screenshot of the "client site" laptop monitor saved during the inaugural first "German" ultrastructural telepathology connection via the Internet between Regensburg and Bochum (May 6, 2000, SCUR-Meeting; approximately 500 km distance). Note the high-resolution "snapshot" image (original magnification ×10,000) displaying a GOM deposit in a dermal blood vessel wall (diagnostic for CADASIL) and the immediately performed size measurement (red parallel lines and the result in the table below). Simple mouse clicks on the buttons visible in the EM-control panel allowed the magnification, beam blanker (on/off), illumination adjustment, control of the stage navigation, and coarse/fine focus adjustment

experience the live remote operation of the EM in Regensburg but also learn interactively how to make the diagnosis of this peculiar disease.

Since 2004, the microscope was retrofitted with a motorized and automatic adjustable special (seven-hole) objective aperture, which was necessary for remote low-magnification range observations (9–2,000×) (to avoid image area clipping by the aperture). In 2006, an additional $1k \times 1k$ fast frame-transfer CCD camera (5 MHz clock) with a fiber-optic-coupled YAG scintillator (TRS'/Moorenweis, Germany) was side-entry mounted to the EM column and USB connected to the server computer (Dell Precision 380, 3.2 GHz Pentium processor, 2 GB internal memory) (Fig. 14.4). This side-entry camera is placed above the fluorescent

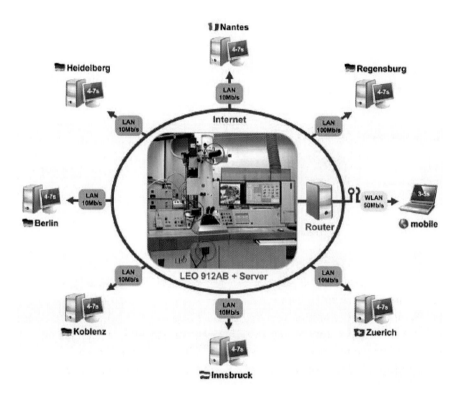

Fig. 14.4. Scheme of the server–client architecture of the electron microscopy telepathology consultation system at the University Regensburg. The LEO912 EFTEM is retrofitted with a motorized drift-minimized objective aperture, and a $1k \times 1k$ pixel CCD camera is bottom- and side-entry-mounted on the EM column (*red encircled*). The system is controlled by a Windows-XP server running the "iTEM" software and handling the communication via standard LAN or WLAN links to the Internet. The image transmission performance of the system in the "live mode" is 1–3 frames per second; in the "frozen snapshot mode" (uncompressed high-resolution 16-bit images for storage) the transfer needs 4–7 s (dependent on daytime bandwidth)

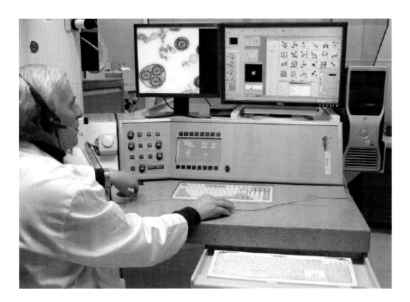

Fig. 14.5. The "server site" operator can flexibly control the EM alternatively by the software button controls and/or conventionally use the microscope panel knobset. The software supports a two-monitor image display; note the left screen showing the live image (abnormal cilia), the large right-hand screen displays the control panels (EM parameters, CCD camera, FFT-Image-Aid, and histogram), the images in the live computer memory, and the currently used database. The telepresence "feeling" in a telepathological consultation can be markedly increased by hooking it up to a parallel standard phone connection (a headset is a helpful tool enabling – here the author – freehand EM operation)

observation screen and is superior to the bottom-mounted camera for tissue-section examinations (comparable to a "wide-angle" lens effect in ordinary photography). The monitors were replaced by large, high-resolution, calibrated, flat-screen TFT monitors to improve the image display and databank handling, while, for the parallel verbal communication with the remote expert during the consultation, a headset for standard phone connection was used (Fig. 14.5).

14.8
Extension of the Server–Client Architecture

In the meantime, the client "analySIS" software (now upgraded by the "iTEM" software package, OSIS/Muenster, Germany; www.olympus-sis.com) was installed on Windows-XP running desktops in different locations (Fig. 14.4): Pathology Innsbruck/Austria, Thomas Mairinger; Pathology Zurich/

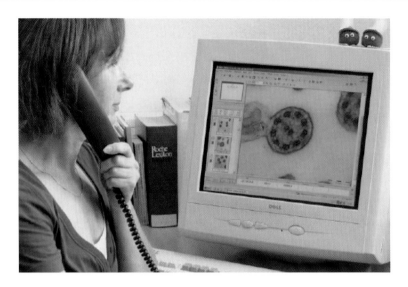

Fig. 14.6. The remote "client site" monitor displaying a transmitted high-resolution 16-bit image from the server and deposited on the local memory computer of the expert (abnormal cilium). Note the overlay discussion tools that can be synchronized with the image from both sites (server = *blue arrow*; remote client/expert = *red arrow*) (Image courtesy of B. Hauroeder, Bundeswehr/Koblenz)

Switzerland, Stefan Kolb; Bundeswehr (Central Institute of the Federal Armed Forces Medical Service) Koblenz/Germany, Baerbel Hauroeder (Fig. 14.6); Laboratoire de Therapie Genetique INCERM U649 Nantes/France, Fabienne Rolling (Fig. 14.7); Dermatology Reference EM-Lab Heidelberg/ Germany, Ingrid Hausser (Fig. 14.8); and Robert-Koch-Institute (National Reference Lab Rapid Virus Diagnosis) Berlin/Germany, Norbert Bannert and Hans Gelderblom for feasibility testing and improvement in the remote EM operation under different Internet bandwidth settings and limitations (ISDN, LAN, ADSL, and WLAN). Since 2004, the server is connected by a 100 Mbps LAN to the Internet, and, for IT security reasons and Firewall restrictions, the clients get access to our server through a VPN channel.

Using the present system configuration, JPEG2000 data compression, and standard client LAN Internet access (10 Mbps), we obtained in the preview "live-image" mode (used for screening the sample; image size 1,024 × 1,024 pixel, 2 MHz pixel-clock at 16 bits, and 100 ms exposure time) at a frame rate of 1–3/s;

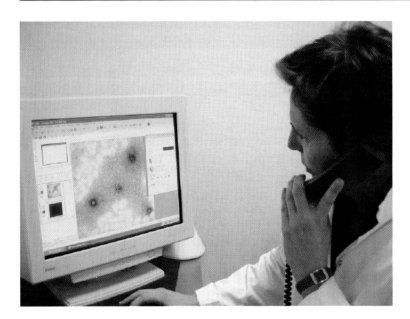

Fig. 14.7. Example of remote basic research consultation of a visual disorder project in collaboration with a French group in Nantes. The quality of the negatively stained recombinant virus particle preparation used in the experimental blindness therapy can be directly assessed on the "client" monitor and commented on through phone by the group leader. (Image courtesy of F. Rolling, Laboratoire de Therapie Genetique, INSERM/Nantes, France)

for the transfer of the uncompressed high-resolution (16 bits, 1,024 × 1,024 pixel) "snapshot" image to the local hard disk, we experienced a transfer time of 4–7 s (depending on date and time of day). During the server–client connection, the remote control capabilities include stage navigation and search for area of interest at low or high resolution in the "live mode," selection of adequate magnification (9–500,000×) in 38 steps, focus adjustment, beam blanker on/ off, illumination intensity adjustment, exposure time setting, and image storage at full resolution (Figs. 14.3 and 14.8). On the "frozen snapshot" high-resolution image overlay, functions like discussion pointer (arrows) and annotation settings or distance measurements are synchronized between the two sites. To increase the telepresence feeling, the live telepathology consultation is usually backed up by a standard phone connection for verbal communication with the remote client/expert.

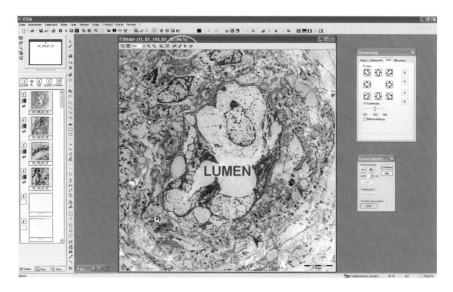

Fig. 14.8. Screenshot of the remote skin ultrastructure expert monitor in Heidelberg consulting a difficult fibrosing lesion in deparaffinized skin tissue of a patient with kidney insufficiency. Teleconference overlay discussion tools (*yellow encircled*: drawing pen, pointing arrows, and annotations) allow the expert to graphically delineate a blood vessel and direct the attention of the observer to important inclusions (*red arrow*); the expert also discusses immediately and by phone the structures pointed out on the server side in Regensburg (*blue arrow*). Note the microscope stage control panel enabling the remote expert to navigate the sample and to decide which section area needs to be examined at higher magnification. (Image courtesy of I. Hausser, Dermatology Department University Hospital/Heidelberg)

14.9
Performance of the Ultrastructural Telepathology

Ultrathin sections of selected diseases (skeletal muscle [minicore disease], skin granuloma [Histiocytosis-X], head tumor [oncocytoma], and skin lesion [Molluscum contagiosum]) as well as negatively stained adeno virus, birna virus, herpes virus, and rotavirus particles were examined remotely and consultation made with the aforementioned experts. The results were presented at the "Ultrapath-XI" Conference of the Society for Ultrastructural Pathology (August 2002, Aspen, CO) and the 15th International Congress on Electron Microscopy in Durban, SA (September 2002). A live ultrastructural telepathology demonstration of the EM examination of poxvirus (Fig. 14.2) and Anthrax spores using wireless Internet access was performed in a special session during the 7th International Conference on the Medical Aspects of Tele-medicine in Regensburg (September 2002) [83]. Mobile expert remote EM operation was also successfully carried out by wireless hotspot Internet access from the airports of Munich/Germany and Denver/USA using, on the client site, a notebook equipped with the Orinoco/Lucent Technology Wireless-PCMCIA-card (maximum 11 Mbps), revealing sufficient performance for the microscope control and only slightly prolonged image transfer in comparison to wired Internet connection. In summer 2006, we performed an outdoor test of the wireless new UMTS communication option (measured mean bandwidth 0.320 Mbps) offered by national telecommunication companies (UMTS PCM-CIA-card, T-Mobile, and Vodafone) (Fig. 14.9). We successfully completed a remote microscope operation and experienced a stable but markedly slower image transfer rate (mean 0.2 fps for "live images" and 130–280 s for high-resolution "snapshots").

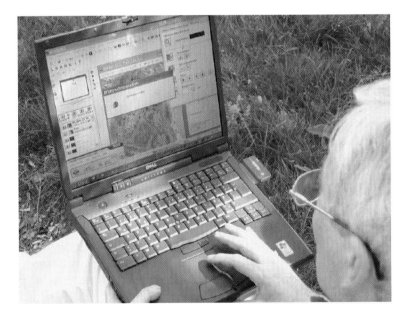

Fig. 14.9. Demonstration of an outdoor wireless remote access on the telepathology system in Regensburg. The "client" expert notebook was equipped with a dedicated UMTS PCMCIA-card (*pink colored*), which uses the new telecommunication channel of T-Mobile and Vodafone company. We experienced stable connections, but the available bandwidth (0.320 Mbps) caused a significant image transfer delay. (UMTS-cards, courtesy of T-Mobile and Vodafone Regensburg)

14.10
Illustrative Telepathology Diagnostic and Basic Research Examples

Recently, a paraffin block containing a skin biopsy from an elderly patient with a suspicion of nephrogenic fibrosing dermopathy (NFD) was referred for EM examination, with special attention on the presence of gadolinium deposits. NFD (also termed NSF, nephrogenic systemic fibrosis) is a painful and disabling recently documented disease observed mainly in patients with renal insufficiency (dialysis or kidney transplant patients) with a previous gadolinium exposure, the etiology of the disease being so far elusive [90]. Gadolinium is a rare-earth element and, owing to its paramagnetic properties, it is widely used as a relatively safe contrast agent in clinical magnetic resonance imaging. The patient concerned had been dialysis-dependent and also had a history of gadolinium exposure; the light microscopy skin histopathology was suggestive for NFD, but other differential diagnoses like autoimmune disorders (such as scleroderma) had to be considered. In the deparaffinized skin sample, we found some tiny perivascular aggregates of undefined material and performed a telepathology "second-opinion" consultation with a skin pathology expert in Heidelberg to exclude possible artifactual findings. The direct telepathologic examination of the sections (choosing different section areas and magnifications) by the expert resulted in an instant confirmation of possible real deposits of inorganic material (Fig. 14.8). This immediately prompted us to perform an in situ elemental analysis using the ESI (electron spectroscopic imaging) and EELS (electron energy loss spectroscopy) methodology with our EFTEM to clear the nature of the deposits in question. This had a considerable impact for the patient's further treatment and is probably also important for the etiologic understanding of the disease [85].

We are cooperating with a French INSERM molecular genetics research group concerning a study of visual disorder in Briard dogs, which are an important animal model for developing a therapy for human blindness caused by hereditary retinal degeneration. After the discovery that a microdeletion mutation in a defined gene (RPE65) is responsible for the disease in dogs and primates, a recombinant vector construct AAV-RPE65 (adeno-associated virus – missing cDNA of the RPE65 gene) was injected subretinally into the affected eyes, and restoration of vision was reported [4,89]. The quality of the AVV-vector particle preparations can be examined by the rapid negative staining procedure and remotely and directly assessed and discussed by all the cooperating participants (Fig. 14.7), saving time and traveling costs.

In rapid viral diagnosis by EM, which is based on the characteristic virus family particle morphology and size, some clinical samples can pose diagnostic difficulties even for experienced investigators. This is a typical situation for a live "second-opinion" request during the daily routine case diagnosis with experts of the Robert-Koch-Institute Reference Laboratory in Berlin and/or the Bundeswehr Medical Centre in Koblenz. The telepresence sample examination and case discussion at the monitor with an expert mostly allow a clear-cut diagnosis and provide significant learning opportunities (for both sides). It is worth noting that the Bundeswehr EM laboratory has similar server telepathology equipment (sibling Zeiss-TEM and TRS-camera, iTEM software) and can provide remote telepathology support (Fig. 14.10).

The concept of remote diagnostic EM was presented to the public in the traditional so-called "Long Night of Science" event (Berlin, 15 June 2002). Numerous visitors of the Robert-Koch-Institute had the opportunity firsthand to remotely operate our TEM in Regensburg and observe different infectious agents (Fig. 14.11).

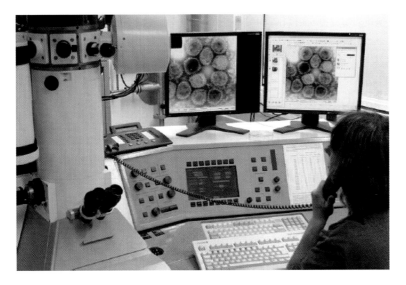

Fig. 14.10. Illustration of the "server site" of the similarly designed and equipped ultrastructural telepathology system of the Bundeswehr's EM laboratory. This is an example of distant teaching: Regensburg was connected as a remote "client" to this system, learning about diagnostic peculiarities in herpes diagnostics. Note the use of discussion tools and the parallel voice support enhancing the telepresence effect for the session participants. (Image courtesy of B. Hauroeder, Bundeswehr/Koblenz)

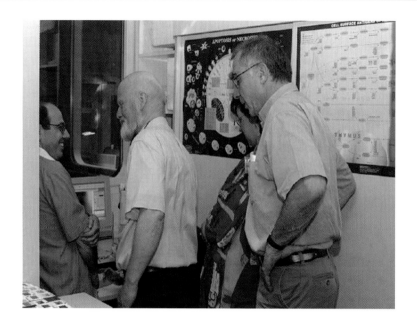

Fig. 14.11. Documentation from the "Long Night of Science" in Berlin, 15 June 2002. Visitors interested in science of the Robert-Koch-Institute got an introduction to telepresence microscopy by H. Gelderblom (second from left) and operated firsthand our EM in Regensburg looking remotely at different infectious agents. (Image courtesy of H. Gelderblom, RKI/ Berlin)

14.11
Discussion and Conclusions

The digital revolution and rapidly expanding telecommunication and computing ability have forced new developments like telepathology and "virtual microscopy" in the light microscopy pathologic practice. Competing immunohistochemical and molecular methods and other factors have tended to supplant EM in many diagnostic fields, but now a resurgence of this proven ancillary diagnostic tool is predicted [29,96]. This provides an opportunity to learn from the experiences collected during the evolution of light telemicroscopy technique – to adapt them or discover other solutions more suitable for the specificity of EM. Also, solutions established in material science and more advanced telediagnostic disciplines like teleradiology (similar black and white image features) [24,86,87] might lead to applications in EM.

Significant savings in time in managing difficult ultrastructural diagnoses are already achieved by sharing and discussing images via e-mail (still image, static telepathology), but reliability is limited. However, for effective EM diagnosis, only an interactive dynamic telepathology system can provide the external expert with the opportunity to select the correct details for an accurate diagnosis and avoid the pitfalls of preselected images. The recently established light microscopic "virtual slide" can indeed be extended to selected sample areas at the ultrastructural level [37,49]; this would probably be applied for electronic teaching using the "virtual microscope" rather than for diagnostic purposes. The "iTEM" software used includes an automated image "stitching" module (MIA, multiple image alignment), but the usability for ultrastructural diagnostic purposes is very limited.

Our national and international ultrastructural telepathology sessions demonstrate that available microscopes can be run remotely by desktop computers or workstations using standard Internet links and can provide a reasonably "smooth" operation of the instruments by "real-time" transmission of images via the Internet. To save bandwidth, the EM needs more automation (speed autofocus, constant illumination brightness at magnification changes, and robotic sample loader [54]). Now almost all EM providers offer an integrated remote operation option for their microscopes; unfortunately, interchangeability is still missing and is a heavy obstacle for collaboration between users of different systems. Depending on the individual need of the user, a range of high-resolution and fast, bottom- or side-entry CCD cameras can be chosen, but, currently for telemicroscopy settings, it is advisable to keep the pixel number of the transferred images as small as possible (camera pixel binning is a helpful adjunct). This limitation will probably be compensated by the rapidly growing Internet speed and bandwidth, as well as improved image compression algorithms in the near future.

The telepresence of an expert is a very effective way of obtaining a second opinion in solving diagnostic or research problems and has significant value for teaching and learning, on both server and client side. The influence of human factors is a very important aspect in establishing such new diagnostic techniques [23,52,59]. Psychological resistance or uncertainty in handling the new tools as well as rendering a diagnosis from a monitor can be a challenge, but this could be compensated by parallel voice assistance and graphic overlay discussion tools. A helpful measure for less experienced users is to hide all but present the only immediately necessary buttons on the graphic user interface. Stepwise and regular training increases familiarity with the system and markedly reduces remote examination time.

Telemicroscopy and the digital image have opened new doors for scientific cooperation, image sharing, consulting, and distant learning, with other microscopy experts. For light microscopy, specialized telediagnosis systems such as those of the AFIP/USA [64,108], UICC-TPCC/Berlin [21,45], and iPATH/ Basel (Internet based on an open telemedicine platform) [8,49] with specific performance have been developed. Now mainly for research purposes, a new kind of cooperation using worldwide-distributed hardware and software resources (nodes) have been linked together, and the so-called Grid technology will be established [5,26,34,60] (the name comes from the electrical power grid that works in a similar manner). This "distributed or parallel computing" uses the Internet as a communication layer and allows access to geographically widespread and sometimes unique resources – for example, dedicated light and electron microscopes, computing performance, information in databases, and services, respecting the rules of the economy of scale (which, e.g., determinate the relation between the size of a plant and the production costs). Different Grids are already established, for example, the Telescience Project at the NCMIR, San Diego, CA, for life science and microscopy [94] and the PRAGMA (Pacific Rim and Grid Middleware Assembly) [74]; the trend may culminate in the development of virtual institutions [48].

No doubt, in the globalized and digitized world of tomorrow and the stepwise population conversion into the "information era," these new cyberspace structures and tools will change the face of future medical care, including pathology [3,65,110]. Old and new diseases and emerging infectious or adverse environmental agents need to be managed by raising costs for resources and energy worldwide. Telemedicine in concert with eScience and eHealth solutions has the potential to offer an efficient health service to everybody independently of geographical location and social status [112]. In trust of this knowledge and vision, we have to work in our subdiscipline of ultrastructural telepathology to establish practical solutions to manage the requirements of modern health-care systems for time and cost reduction [9,18,49] while maintaining the highest diagnostic standards. The telepathology motto, "move the image, not the patient," will help to direct us to achieve these objectives.

14.12
Summary

- Electron microscopy – owing to its high-resolution power – can provide significant data at the ultrastructural level in tissue-based pathological diagnosis. In some subspecialties (kidney, skin, and ciliary disorders) EM is indispensable; virus diagnosis can be rendered with unprecedented speed.
- In 1999, we established an Internet-based interactive dynamic telepathology system combining remote operation of an EM, digital image acquisition, and software specifically tailored for collaborative needs.
- Remote experts can examine samples directly with adequate EM functionality, and, in case of diagnostic dilemmas, the consulting "second-opinion" expert is no longer constrained by problems inherent in preselected images.

- We demonstrated that the ultrastructural telepathology system can be remotely operated using standard workstations and Internet connections with experts in different localities; together with teleconferencing tools it provides increased effectiveness and support for diagnosis, research, and distant teaching.
- Further progress in EM automation and growing Internet bandwidth will foster such interactive telemicroscopy solutions and, through implementation into the developing Grid technology, enable new collaborative opportunities, saving time and resources.

Acknowledgements

The author acknowledges the technical support of Beate Voll and Heiko Siegmund/Regensburg, as well as linguistic help from Brian Eyden/Manchester,UK

References

1. Aas IH (2002) Changes in the job situation due to telemedicine. J Telemed Telecare 8(1):41–47
2. Aas IH (2002) Learning in organizations working with telemedicine. J Telemed Telecare 8(2):107–111
3. Aas IH (2002) Telemedicine and changes in the distribution of tasks between levels of care. J Telemed Telecare 8(Suppl 2):1–2
4. Acland GM, Aguirre GD, Ray J, et al. (2001) Gene therapy restores vision in a canine model of childhood blindness. Nat Genet 28(1):92–95
5. Akiyama T, Teranishi Y, Nozaki K, et al. (2005) Scientific grid activities and PKI deployment in the Cybermedia Center, Osaka University. J Clin Monit Comput 19(4–5):279–294
6. Baak JP, van Diest PJ, Meijer GA (2000) Experience with a dynamic inexpensive videoconferencing system for frozen section telepathology. Anal Cell Pathol 21(3–4): 169–175
7. Boutonnat J, Paulin C, Faure C, Colle PE, Ronot X, Seigneurin D (2006) A pilot study in two French medical schools for teaching histology using virtual microscopy. Morphologie 90(288):21–25
8. Brauchli K, Oberholzer M (2005) The iPath telemedicine platform. J Telemed Telecare 11(Suppl 2):S3–S7
9. Bryant J (2000) Cost minization analysis of telepathology: a critical review. Am J Clin Pathol 113(6):902–905
10. Buzug TM, Handels H, Holz D (2001) Telemedicine: medicine and communication. Kluwer, New York
11. Coiera E (1997) Guide to medical informatics, the Internet, and telemedicine, 1st edn. Chapman & Hall Medical, London
12. Coma de Corral MJ, Pena HJ (1999) Quo vadis telemedicine? Rev Neurol 29(5):478–483
13. Dalla Palma P, Morelli L, Forti S, et al. (2001) Telemetric intraoperative diagnosis among hospitals in Trentino: first evaluations and optimization of the procedure. Pathologica 93(1):34–38

14. Dawson PJ, Johnson JG, Edgemon LJ, Brand CR, Hall E, Van Buskirk GF (2000) Outpatient frozen sections by telepathology in a veterans administration medical center. Hum Pathol 31(7):786–788

15. Della Mea V, Cataldi P, Pertoldi B, Beltrami CA (1999) Dynamic robotic telepathology: a preliminary evaluation on frozen sections, histology and cytology. J Telemed Telecare 5(Suppl 1):S55–S56

16. Della Mea V, Roberto V, Conti A, di Gaspero L, Beltrami CA (1999) Internet agents for telemedicine services. Med Inform Internet Med 24(3):181–188

17. Della Mea V, Cataldi P, Pertoldi B, Beltrami CA (2000) Combining dynamic and static robotic telepathology: a report on 184 consecutive cases of frozen sections, histology and cytology. Anal Cell Pathol 20(1):33–39

18. Della Mea V, Cortolezzis D, Beltrami CA (2000) The economics of telepathology – a case study. J Telemed Telecare 6(Suppl 1):S168–S169

19. Demichelis F, Barbareschi M, Dalla Palma P, Forti S (2002) The virtual case: a new method to completely digitize cytological and histological slides. Virchows Arch 441(2):159–164

20. Dickersin GR (2000) Diagnostic electron microscopy: a text/atlas, 2nd edn. Springer, New York

21. Dietel M, Nguyen-Dobinsky TN, Hufnagl P (2000) The UICC Telepathology Consultation Center. International Union against Cancer. A global approach to improving consultation for pathologists in cancer diagnosis. Cancer 89(1):187–191

22. Dolled-Filhart M, Ryden L, Cregger M, et al. (2006) Classification of breast cancer using genetic algorithms and tissue microarrays. Clin Cancer Res 12(21):6459–6468

23. Draper JV, Kaber DB, Usher JM (1998) Telepresence. Hum Factors 40(3):354–375

24. Dreyer KJ (2006) PACS: a guide to the digital revolution, 2nd edn. Springer, New York

25. Dykstra MJ, Reuss LE (2003) Biological electron microscopy. Theory, techniques, and troubleshooting, 2nd edn. Kluwer, New York

26. EGEE (2008) Enabling grids for E-Science. http://www.eu-egee.org/

27. Elles R, Mountford R (2004) Molecular diagnosis of genetic diseases, 2nd edn. Humana Press, Totowa, NJ

28. Erlandson RA (1994) Diagnostic transmission electron microscopy of tumors: with clinicopathological, immunohistochemical, and cytogenetic correlations. Raven Press, New York

29. Erlandson RA (2003) Role of electron microscopy in modern diagnostic surgical pathology. In: Cote W, Weiss S (eds) Modern surgical pathology. Saunders, Philadelphia, PA

30. Erlandson RA, Rosai J (1995) A realistic approach to the use of electron microscopy and other ancillary diagnostic techniques in surgical pathology. Am J Surg Pathol 19(3):247–250

31. Eyden B (1996) Organelles in tumor diagnosis: an ultrastructural atlas. Igaku-Shoin, New York

32. Eyden B (1999) Electron microscopy in tumour diagnosis: continuing to complement other diagnostic techniques. Histopathology 35(2):102–108

33. Ferrer-Roca O, Sosa-Iudicissa MC (1998) Handbook of telemedicine. IOS Press, Amsterdam, Washington DC

34. Foster I, Kesselman C (2004) The grid: blueprint for a new computing infrastructure, 2nd edn. Morgan Kaufmann, Amsterdam, Boston

35. Ghadially FN (1997) Ultrastructural pathology of the cell and matrix, 4th edn. Butterworth-Heinemann, Boston

36. Goldsmith CS, Tatti KM, Ksiazek TG, et al. (2004) Ultrastructural characterization of SARS coronavirus. Emerg Infect Dis 10(2):320–326

37. Gu J, Ogilvie RW (2005) Virtual microscopy and virtual slides in teaching, diagnosis, and research. Taylor & Francis, Boca Raton

38. Hadida-Hassan M, Young SJ, Peltier ST, Wong M, Lamont S, Ellisman MH (1999) Web-based telemicroscopy. J Struct Biol 125(2–3):235–245

39. Hagens v.G (2007) Body Worlds. http://www.bodyworlds.com/en.html

40. Haroske G, Giroud F, Kunze KD, Meyer W (2000) A telepathology based virtual reference and certification centre for DNA image cytometry. Anal Cell Pathol 21(3–4): 149–159

41. Hazelton PR, Gelderblom HR (2003) Electron microscopy for rapid diagnosis of infectious agents in emergent situations. Emerg Infect Dis 9(3):294–303

42. Herrera GA, Lowery MC, Turbat-Herrera EA (2000) Immunoelectron microscopy in the age of molecular pathology. Appl Immunohistochem Mol Morphol 8(2):87–97

43. Hufnagl P, Bayer G, Oberbamscheidt P, et al. (2000) Comparison of different telepathology solutions for primary frozen section diagnostic. Anal Cell Pathol 21(3–4):161–167

44. Hutarew G, Schlicker HU, Idriceanu C, Strasser F, Dietze O (2006) Four years experience with teleneuropathology. J Telemed Telecare 12(8):387–391

45. Kayser K (2002) Interdisciplinary telecommunication and expert teleconsultation in diagnostic pathology: present status and future prospects. J Telemed Telecare 8(6):325–330

46. Kayser K, Szymas J, Weinstein RS (1999) Telepathology: telecommunication, electronic education, and publication in pathology. Springer, Berlin, New York

47. Kayser K, Beyer M, Blum S, Kayser G (2000) Telecommunication – a new tool for quality assurance and control in diagnostic pathology. Folia Neuropathol 38(2):79–83

48. Kayser K, Kayser G, Radziszowski D, Oehmann A (2004) New developments in digital pathology: from telepathology to virtual pathology laboratory. Stud Health Technol Inform 105:61–69

49. Kayser K, Molnar B, Weinstein RS (2006) Virtual microscopy. VSV Interdisciplinary Medical Publishing, Berlin

50. Kok LP, Boon ME (2003) Microwaves for the art of microscopy. Coulomb Press Leyden, Leiden

51. Kricka LJ, Fortina P (2001) Microarray technology and applications: an all-language literature survey including books and patents. Clin Chem 47(8):1479–1482

52. Krupinski EA, Tillack AA, Richter L, et al. (2006) Eye-movement study and human performance using telepathology virtual slides: implications for medical education and differences with experience. Hum Pathol 37(12):1543–1556

53. Kumar RK, Freeman B, Velan GM, De Permentier PJ (2006) Integrating histology and histopathology teaching in practical classes using virtual slides. Anat Rec B New Anat 289(4):128–133

54. Lefman J, Morrison R, Subramaniam S (2007) Automated 100-position specimen loader and image acquisition system for transmission electron microscopy. J Struct Biol 158(3):318–326

55. Leong AS, Visinoni F, Visinoni C, Milios J (2000) An advanced digital image-capture computer system for gross specimens: a substitute for gross description. Pathology 32(2):131–135

56. Linderoth HC (2002) Managing telemedicine: from noble ideas to action. J Telemed Telecare 8(3):143–150

57. Madeley CR (2003) Diagnosing smallpox in possible bioterrorist attack. Lancet 361(9352):97–98

58. Madeley CR, Field AM (1998) Virus morphology, 2nd edn. Churchill Livingstone, Edinburgh, New York

59. Mairinger T (2000) Acceptance of telepathology in daily practice. Anal Cell Pathol 21 (3–4):135–140

60. Martone ME, Gupta A, Ellisman MH (2004) E-neuroscience: challenges and triumphs in integrating distributed data from molecules to brains. Nat Neurosci 7(5):467–472

61. Mierau GW (1999) Electron microscopy for tumour diagnosis: is it redundant? Histopathology 35(2):99–101

62. Miller SE (2003) Bioterrorism and electron microscopic differentiation of poxviruses from herpesviruses: dos and don'ts. Ultrastruct Pathol 27(3):133–140

63. Morens DM, Folkers GK, Fauci AS (2004) The challenge of emerging and re-emerging infectious diseases. Nature 430(6996):242–249

64. Mullick FG, Fontelo P, Pemble C (1996) Telemedicine and telepathology at the Armed Forces Institute of Pathology: history and current mission. Telemed J 2(3):187–193

65. Murphy WM (2007) Anatomical pathology in the 21st century: the great paradigm shift. Hum Pathol 38(7):957–962

66. Nagata H, Mizushima H (1998) World wide microscope: new concept of internet telepathology microscope and implementation of the prototype. Medinfo 9(Pt 1):286–289

67. NASA (2004) Mars exploration rover mission. http://marsrovers.jpl.nasa.gov/newsroom/ pressreleases/20040305a.html

68. Onguru O, Celasun B (2000) Intra-hospital use of a telepathology system. Pathol Oncol Res 6(3):197–201

69. Ordonez NG, Mackay B (1998) Electron microscopy in tumor diagnosis: indications for its use in the immunohistochemical era. Hum Pathol 29(12):1403–1411

70. Papadimitriou JM, Henderson DW, Spagnolo DV (1992) Diagnostic ultrastructure of non-neoplastic diseases. Churchill Livingstone, Edinburgh, New York

71. Perkins JM, Blom DA, McComb DW, Allard LF (2007) Functional remote microscopy via the AtlanTICC Alliance. Microsc Microanal 13(Suppl 2):1702–1703

72. Petersen I, Wolf G, Roth K, Schluns K (2000) Telepathology by the Internet. J Pathol 191(1):8–14

73. Picot J (2000) Meeting the need for educational standards in the practice of telemedicine and telehealth. J Telemed Telecare 6(Suppl 2):S59–S62

74. PRAGMA (2006) Pacific rim applications and grid middleware assembly. http://www. pragma-grid.net/

75. Ranchod M (2003) Intraoperative consultations in surgical pathology. In: Cote W, Weiss S (eds) Modern surgical pathology. Saunders, Philadelphia, PA

76. Rashbass J (2000) The impact of information technology on histopathology. Histopathology 36(1):1–7

77. Rembrandt vR (1632) The Anatomy Lesson of Dr. Tulp. http://www.sgipt.org/kunst/ medizin/sektion

78. Sambrook J, Russell DW (2001) Molecular cloning: a laboratory manual, 3rd edn. Cold Spring Harbor Laboratory Press, Cold Spring Harbor, NY

79. Sawai T, Uzuki M, Watanabe M (2000) Telepathology at presence and in the future. Rinsho Byori 48(5):458–462

80. Schlag PM (1997) On the way to new horizons: telemedicine in oncology. Oncologist 2(2):III–IV

81. Schroeder JA, Voelkl E (1998) Electron microscopy examination of pathological samples in Oak Ridge/USA by remote control via Internet from Regensburg/Germany: a live ultrastructure-telepathology presentation. Abstracts G7SP4 Conference: the impact of telemedicine on health care management, Regensburg, Germany 1998:84

82. Schroeder JA, Voelkl E, Hofstaedter F (2001) Ultrastructural telepathology – remote EM-diagnostic via Internet. Ultrastruct Pathol 25(4):301–307

83. Schroeder JA, Voelkl E, Hofstaedter F (2002) Ultrastructural telepathology – an application of remote electron microscopy via Internet. Eur J Med Res 7(Suppl 1):74–75

84. Schroeder JA, Gelderblom HR, Hauroeder B, Schmetz C, Milios J, Hofstaedter F (2006) Microwave-assisted tissue processing for same-day EM-diagnosis of potential bioterrorism and clinical samples. Micron 37(6):577–590

85. Schroeder JA, Weingart C, Coras B, et al. (2008) Ultrastructural evidence of dermal gadolinium deposits in a patient with nephrogenic systemic fibrosis and end-stage renal disease. Clin J Am Soc Nephrol 3(4):968–975

86. Seiwerth S, Danilovic Z (2000) The telepathology and teleradiology network in Croatia. Anal Cell Pathol 21(3–4):223–228

87. Siegel EL, Kolodner RM (1999) Filmless radiology. Springer, New York

88. Stanberry B (2000) Telemedicine: barriers and opportunities in the 21st century. J Intern Med 247(6):615–628

89. Stieger K, Mendes-Madeira A, Meur GL, et al. (2007) Oral administration of doxycycline allows tight control of transgene expression: a key step towards gene therapy of retinal diseases. Gene Ther 14(23):1668–1673

90. Swaminathan S, Shah SV (2007) New insights into nephrogenic systemic fibrosis. J Am Soc Nephrol 18(10):2636–2643

91. Szymas J, Wolf G (1999) Remote microscopy through the internet. Pol J Pathol 50(1):37–42

92. Szymas J, Papierz W, Danilewicz M (2000) Real-time teleneuropathology for a second opinion of neurooncological cases. Folia Neuropathol 38(1):43–46

93. Takaoka A, Yoshida K, Mori H, Hayashi S, Young SJ, Ellisman MH (2000) International telemicroscopy with a 3 MV ultrahigh voltage electron microscope. Ultramicroscopy 83(1–2):93–101

94. Telescience Project (2006) http://ncmir.ucsd.edu/

95. Tucker JA (2000) The continuing value of electron microscopy in surgical pathology. Ultrastruct Pathol 24(6):383–389

96. Turbat-Herrera EA, D'Agostino H, Herrera GA (2004) The use of electron microscopy to refine diagnoses in the daily practice of cytopathology. Ultrastruct Pathol 28(2):55–66

97. Ultrastructural Telepathology - EM Diagnostic via Internet (2000) SCUR 2000 Meeting: histo-morphology, today and tomorrow. Bochum, Germany

98. Virchow RLK (1858) Die cellularpathologie in ihrer begründung auf physiologische und pathologische gewebelehre. A. Hirschwald, Berlin

99. Voelkl E, Allard LF, Nolan TA, Hill D, Lehman M (1997) Remote operation of electron microscopes. Scanning 19:286–291

100. Walter GF, Matthies HK, Brandis A, von Jan U (2000) Telemedicine of the future: teleneuropathology. Technol Health Care 8(1):25–34

101. Weidner N (2003) Modern surgical pathology. 1st ed. Saunders, Philadelphia

102. Weinstein RS, Bloom KJ, Rozek LS (1987) Telepathology and the networking of pathology diagnostic services. Arch Pathol Lab Med 111(7):646–652

103. Weinstein RS, Bhattacharyya A, Yu YP, et al. (1995) Pathology consultation services via the Arizona-International Telemedicine Network. Arch Anat Cytol Pathol 43(4):219–226

104. Weinstein RS, Bhattacharyya AK, Graham AR, Davis JR (1997) Telepathology: a ten-year progress report. Hum Pathol 28(1):1–7

105. Weinstein RS, Descour MR, Liang C, et al. (2001) Telepathology overview: from concept to implementation. Hum Pathol 32(12):1283–1299

106. Wellnitz U, Binder B, Fritz P, Friedel G, Schwarzmann P (2000) Reliability of telepathology for frozen section service. Anal Cell Pathol 21(3–4):213–222

107. Wells CA, Sowter C (2000) Telepathology: a diagnostic tool for the millennium? J Pathol 191(1):1–7

108. Williams BH, Mullick FG, Butler DR, Herring RF, O'Leary TJ (2001) Clinical evaluation of an international static image-based telepathology service. Hum Pathol 32(12):1309–1317

109. Winokur TS, McClellan S, Siegal GP, et al. (2000) A prospective trial of telepathology for intraoperative consultation (frozen sections). Hum Pathol 31(7):781–785

110. Wootton R (2006) Realtime telemedicine. J Telemed Telecare 12(7):328–336

111. Wright M (1999) Publication of the Material Microcharacterisation Collaboratory ORNL. http://www.ornl.gov/sci/doe2k/MICSReview/99/publications.html

112. Yogesan K (2006) Teleophthalmology. Springer, Berlin, New York

113. Zaluzec NJ (1998) Tele-presence microscopy: a progress Report. Microsc Microanal 4(Suppl 2):18–19

114. Zaluzec NJ (2007) TelePresence Microscopy Collaboratory. http://tpm.amc.anl.gov/

115. Zhou J, Hogarth MA, Walters RF, Green R, Nesbitt TS (2000) Hybrid system for telepathology. Hum Pathol 31(7):829–833

Remote Control of the Scanning Electron Microscope

Atsushi Yamada

15.1
Scanning Electron Microscope

First, a scanning electron microscope (SEM) is described briefly.

15.1.1
Principle

An SEM uses an electron beam that is shorter than the wavelength of light. The electron beam is focused on a specimen. A detector detects the secondary and the backscattered electrons, which are emitted from a specimen, and these reflect the surface shape of a specimen on an observation display as an image signal (Fig. 15.1). The SEM image shows that the depth of focus to be more compared with an optical microscope. We can observe a sample to magnify the surface structure in three dimensions, same mechanism as in human eyes (Photo1: example of image/calcarina). An operator can find the observation point easily at low magnification, even if unevenness is shown on the sample surface. An SEM can magnify the specimen surface image from 10 to 1 million times and one can observe detailed structure close at hand.

15.1.2
Treatment of Biological Sample

As for the SEM, a specimen chamber is evacuated to use an electron beam. Since a biological sample has moisture content, it does not have sufficient conductivity. So the sample needs processing.

1. The biological sample including the water protein was fixed chemically and the sample was dried using chemicals so that it does not change when put

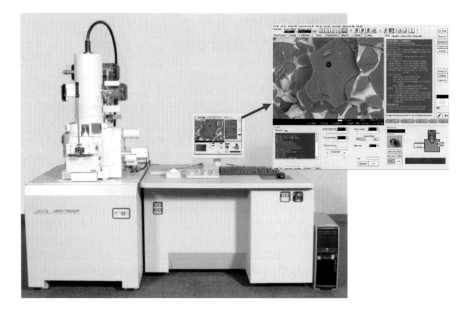

Fig. 15.1. Scanning electron microscope (JAM-7500F:JEOL). A scanning electron microscope (SEM) uses an electron beam that is shorter than the wavelength of light source

in vacuum. The processed sample is fixed to a sample holder with special adhesives.

2. The biological sample does not have conductivity. Therefore, when electron beam scans the sample, the electron collects on the sample surface and the sample is charged up.

For this reason, we must coat the surface of the sample with gold or platinum or palladium (this improves the efficiency of the secondary electron signal generated from a sample), in order to improve prevention of the charge accumulation and the quality of image. In the case of a biological sample, such treatment is necessary. A specialist processes the sample when an SEM operator doesn't know the method of the sample production. And the operator needs to set the treated sample to the specimen chamber of SEM immediately to prevent the contamination of the sample.

15.1.3
Observation

An operator sets the pretreated sample to SEM, irradiates the sample with an electron beam, adjusts a focus, and observes an image. As for the recent SEM, image processor technology develops rapidly, and the general person is able to observe high-magnification images. In the same way in an optical microscope, the operator can observe the image only by moving the SEM to the position that is to be observed and setting the focus.

15.2
Remote Control of the SEM

15.2.1
Effectiveness of the Remote Control

The remote control properties of the SEM can be used for academic training and for communication between a laboratory and a factory, besides telepathology. An SEM operator and an observer at a remote place share the same information through the live image of a real sample at the same time. For example, a doctor sends a sample to a main hospital having an SEM, and a specialist treats the sample accordingly. An operator sets the sample to the SEM. The doctor who sent the sample and the pathologist then observe the image of the sample surface and try to analyze it together. However, the hospital in spite of having an SEM may not have a pathologist from the same field. In this case, the most suitable pathologist participates from other hospitals and university, and a doctor can advice on the particular problem. Even if the pathologist is not present at the place where SEM was installed, SEM operation of the actual image can be carried out from a remote place. Thus, efficient work is possible. Considering the limited number of SEMs and the pathologists available, the remote control using the Internet that covers the whole world is a very effective system. Furthermore, it is also possible to share information and improve the efficiency of the whole work by maintaining databases containing observation/analysis results. Remote control of SEM is very effective in pathological diagnosis; it extends the concept of telepathology further and is expected to help in advanced medical diagnosis.

15.2.2
Conditions Required For Remote Control

To operate SEM by remote control from various places, the following conditions are needed.
SEM connection:

1. Be in the environment where SEM can be connected through LAN/Internet.
2. SEM is having integrated control protocol for enabling communication with Client PC.
3. The live image should be transferred to LAN/Internet as a digital image.

Environment of an external client:

1. External client PCs does not need special hardware and software.
2. The bandwidth required for transmission and control of an SEM image is secured.

Communication function:

1. The communication function of the Net-meeting etc. should be able to be used together.

Remote control operation of SEM is attained by fulfilling these requirements.

SEM can facilitate communication between the SEM and the client side. As both doctors can discuss the instruction and the sample at the observation position, while observing the same image, the communication can thus be improved.

15.3
Practical Use of Remote Control Lock System

The remote system is divided into two types depending on the structure of the SEM.

1. System using a web browser: The system equipped with the image display and the SEM control function on the general web browser.
2. Remote desktop system: A method to display observation screen of SEM to external client.

These two systems differ depending on the structure of SEM. Each system is explained further.

15.3.1
System Using a Web Browser

The system using a web browser is applicable to SEM generally used widely at present. This system is realizable if SEM has a signal output of the NTSC, which is the standard of a general image output signal, and the external control command of SEM is prepared. We have named this remote control system "WEB-SEM," because this system supports the Internet and has been constructed on a web browser.

15.3.1.1
Construction

Figure 15.2 shows a diagram of the system configuration in which an SEM is connected to the LAN/Internet and controlled from a client PC. The basic unit of an SEM is used as the server, and a PC to perform the remote control of SEM is used as the client PC. The operation system used in the client PC is Windows, because this is a standard OS (we have used Windows XPTM for the WEB-SEM). The SEM is connected to a video server for transmitting live images and is also connected directly to the LAN to allow communication between the SEM and the client PC. The interface for SEM control is displayed on the web browser on the client PC, as shown in Fig. 15.3. The user interface consists basically of an SEM image display and an SEM control part. At the server side, it is necessary to add hardware to the standard SEM for image transmission and communication, although the client PC side does not need any special hardware. Therefore, there is no need to provide any special software in advance, if the client PC is already connected to the network.

15.3.1.2
Communication Method

Figure 15.4 shows the contents of signals for communication between the SEM (server) and the client PC.

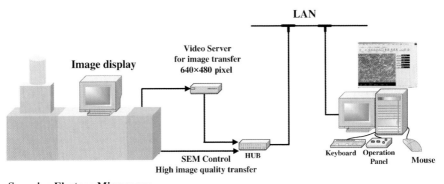

Scanning Electron Microscope   **Client PC**

Fig. 15.2. Block diagram of WEB-SEM remote control system. The SEM is connected to a video server for transferring live images and also connected directly to the LAN to permit communication between the SEM and the client PC. At the SEM (server) side hardware is added to the standard SEM for image transfer and communication. The client side does not need any special software

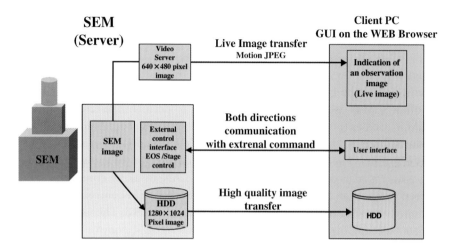

Fig. 15.3. The block diagram of WEB-SEM system communication.
Live image transfer: 640X480/320X240 pixels image transferred by Motion JPEG
Communications: SEM control with external control
Save image transfer: High quality image is saved in the SEM HDD and transferred to the client PC HDD

Live Image

The SEM image transmits the image signal that outputs NTSC to LAN with the video server. The image signals are connected to the video server intended exclusively for the image transfer, and the image is transferred from the video server to the client PC via the LAN. The video server uses an image format of motion JPEG and transfers the images to the LAN using TCP/IP. The transferred images are displayed on the Internet explorer, which is a commonly used web browser in Windows.

SEM Control

A doctor (client PC side) performs a magnification, etc., on the observation screen. Client PC sends a command to control the SEM, such as change a magnification. The host computer attached to the SEM receives this command through Internet and interface part of the external control. Then the client computer changes the hardware of SEM. All the data indicating the instrument statuses are reported to both the host and client computers, so that indication of parameters of both computers is always the same, even if the control was made through either computer.

Image Saving

WEB-SEM transmits a 640 × 480-pixel image as a live image, in order to carry out image observation. However, to enable observation with higher definition, the image must consist of about 1,280 × 960 pixels. In this case, a high-definition image is saved by another method without using the image of a video server. When the operator performs the image-saving operations from the client PC, a high-definition image is saved in the hard disk on the SEM side, and then it is automatically transferred to and saved in the client PC. A high-definition image is automatically saved in the client PC when the operator at the client PC simply specifies the Save button. By this technique, a high-definition image is not dependent on the speed of the line to connect and can certainly be saved. Thus, it is possible to observe a live image and also acquire a high-definition saved image with comfortable operation.

Operation

The method of operating the user interface is described further. An operator starts a web browser on client PC and starts to connect the SEM and the client. After the connection is achieved, the user interface shown in Fig. 15.4

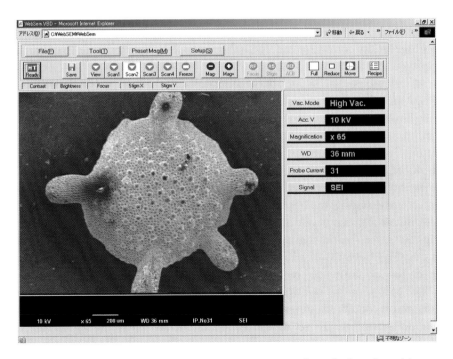

Fig. 15.4. Graphical user interface to WEB-SEM. A user interface is built on the web browser using SEM GUI and can be controlled by a mouse operation alone

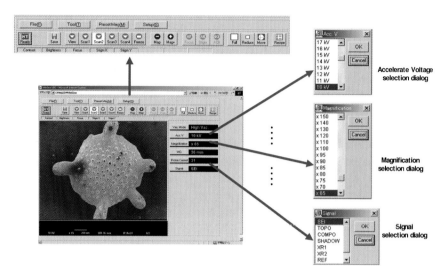

Fig. 15.5. The user interface for operation and the setup button. The operation button is arranged in the top. The setup button is arranged in the right side

is displayed on a web browser. An SEM image, an SEM control button, and an observation condition are displayed on a web browser. The live image displayed on the client PC consists of 640 × 480 pixels, which is sufficient for the observation or the image adjustment (such as focusing). It is roughly classified into button operations and dragging operations using the mouse. Figure 15.5 shows the setup buttons for column, image adjustment, and observation conditions. The menu part has an image-saving button, scanning-speed select buttons, an image-freeze ON/OFF button, magnification select buttons, and autofunction buttons. The feature of these buttons is to be able to execute a series of operation by a single action. These buttons can easily execute an easy switch of the setting, the observation condition setting of the recipe selection, etc. Under the group of button, there are manual control buttons to change the brightness, focus, and stigmator controls. This GUI features a configuration that enables the SEM to be controlled by the mouse operation alone. These button functions are used mainly for controlling the live image.

The button on the right-hand side of an image is used for determining the observation conditions. If observation conditions are known beforehand, these conditions can be easily set up using the aforementioned recipe button. If the observation condition is required to be changed for the sample newly observed, these buttons can be used. You can choose a detector such as SEI (secondary electron image), TOPO (backscattered topography electron image), and COMPO (backscattered composition electron image) for this purpose.

15.3.2
Remote Desktop System

A remote desktop system projects the display on the screen of SEM-side PC (on the image memory of PC) on clients PC screen as it is. This system is represented by the remote desktop of Windows XP and can also simplify connection with LAN/Internet to a great extent.

15.3.2.1
Construction

Figure 15.6 shows the block diagram of a remote desktop system. SEM and client PC are connected to LAN. The software for controlling by a remote desktop is installed in each PC. This control software displays the image data and control display that were developed on PC memory of SEM on a client PC screen. For this reason, the observation screen of SEM displayed on client PC needs to have the function in which SEM is controllable with a mouse. Moreover, the image data need to expand the image on PC memory of an SEM. The conventional SEM has included the image-processing board in the PC to display the special image signal of the SEM image, which consists of the signal of a secondary electron and a backscattered electron on PC screen. In this case, the screen display of SEM is displayed on an observation screen, combining the image developed

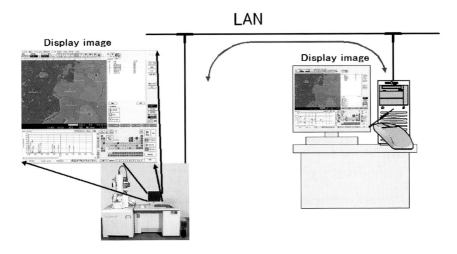

Fig. 15.6. The block diagram of remote desktop. A Client PC displays the SEM observation screen as it is, and controls a SEM from a client PC screen. When the data transmission speeds keep over 5Mbps, an operator can do SEM operation since the image of refresh speed obtains over 5 sheets per second

in the memory of the image-processing board and the control screen built in the memory of the PC. Since an SEM image signal is not expanded on PC memory, an image is not displayed on a client PC screen. Cautions are required (it is necessary to correspond by a WEB-SEM system). The SEM controlled by this system must be to use the type that expands a control display and an image signal display on the memory of PC.

15.3.2.2
Communication Method

To communicate to remote desktop, software installed included Windows XP or a remote system, for example, PCAnywhereTM, made by Symantec into both SEM PC and client. This is a communication method using a remote desktop protocol. The image display extended on PC memory by SEM (server) is transmitted via LAN/Internet and is displayed on a client PC screen as it is. Therefore, a live image display and SEM control are realizable only by remote desktop software. When using for pathology diagnosis, it is effective to choose the remote software that can be operated on both the SEM and the client sides.

Operation

The screen on client PC becomes the same image as the screen display of SEM. For this reason, a client can operate not only an image display but also SEM control like original SEM. The explanation here uses JSM-7500F (product made from JEOL) corresponding to a remote desktop. The display size of JSM-7500F is 1,280 × 1,024 pixels, and the SEM image is displayed at 800 × 600 pixels. The control part of SEM is displayed on portions other than an image display. The operation screen not only can set up observation conditions but also has included the manual operation for a focus or brightness adjustment into the screen display like WEB-SEM. As the SEM can carry out SEM control only in mouse operation, it can also operate a remote desktop as it is from client PC.

15.4
Data Transfer and Response

Remote control is connected to LAN, an exclusive line, and the Internet currently used in general. When connecting client PC with SEM by one-to-one relation (LAN and an exclusive line that restricted the client), it is satisfactory to bandwidth required for remote control and operation. Under the actual operation, the system performance is greatly affected by the extent to which the LAN is congested (the number of line that can be used). In particular, when the connected circuit is crowded, the bandwidth that can be used becomes narrow, and a remote control is not obtained at a sufficiently quick transmission speed. If a communication line is crowded, the response of communication and image transmission will also be slow (refresh rate becomes slow by the client PC). When performing normal observation, it is necessary to refresh the image at the rate of five frames per second to permit stage shift and focusing. SEM must also be smoothly controllable in such a situation. The amount of data transfer and response for remote control are described later.

15.4.1
Amount of Data Transfer

15.4.1.1
WEB-SEM

The amount of data transfer that is needed in WEB-SEM is shown. The data of WEB-SEM are roughly divided into operation protocol and image data. The control signals are used for command-level communication, and so the amount of transferred data is extremely small. On the contrary, the image data account for most of the data transferred to and from WEB-SEM. Motion JPEG was used as the image output format, and the image was transferred using TCP/IP. Because motion JPEG is a method recorded compressing the image of each frame in JPEG, and continuously, the amount of the data transfer is predictable regardless of the display of the image. Figure 15.7 shows an example of the amount of image data used in the case of WEB-SEM. Here, when performing normal observation, refresh speed are defined in the image at the rate of five frames per second to permit stage shift and focusing. The abscissa indicates the image compression ratio, and the ordinate does the amount of image data transferred. The amount of transferred data varies according to the degree of image compression. The video server used here enables the high-definition image to be observed with little degradation (the image becomes a blocked state) due to compression, provided that the image compression rate is weaker than the compression rate represented by line A in Fig. 15.7. To obtain an image-refreshing rate of five frames per second with the use of 640×480-pixel display format, the data transfer speed of about 2 Mbps is necessary.

15.4.1.2
Remote Desktop

The system of a remote desktop transmits an observation screen display to client PC as it is. The amount of the data transfer of this method depends on the size of the display. Especially, the amount of the data transfers increases

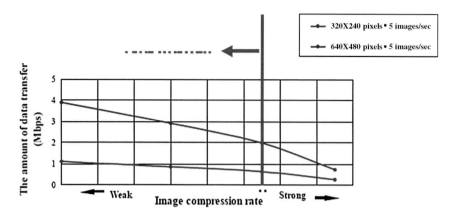

Fig. 15.7. Amount of data transfer: live image (direct connection of SEM and client PC). Image quality becomes worse in the right region of line A. Five images (refresh time) is enough to adjust SEM image

to the image of the scanning microscope, because the entire image is always changing with movement and noise of an image. When the remote system (PCAnywhereTM: made by Symantec) on the market whose operation is possible in both directions by an SEM and a client is used, the amount of data transfer of about 5 Mbps is required. (The setting conditions of software: display size 1,280 × 1,024 pixels, video quality 100.)

15.4.2
Technique for Improving a Response

When operating SEM by remote control via LAN and the Internet, a transmit line becomes congested and sufficient bandwidth is no longer obtained. If the LAN becomes congested, a delay in communication will occur, and also the response delay will take place in control signals sent from the client PC for operating the SEM, such as those for refreshing the image and focusing. When such a delay occurs, a response to the change in the image for the SEM operation slows down, making the system extremely difficult to use. In such a case, a device is needed to operate remote control comfortably. To put it concretely, to operate by remote control, (1) reduction of the amount of the communication data and (2) single action operation in which it is not influenced by the response of a picture are needed. As mentioned above, most communication data is occupied by image data. For example, WEB-SEM is connected to 10 base-T or larger LAN. If the bandwidth more than 2 Mbps is secured, WEB-SEM does not adversely affect the operation. If the line is congested and the communication speed fewer than 2 Mbps can be obtained, the image-refreshing rate will become low. To adapt to such conditions, where it is not possible to secure the data capacity, we show the method to perform smooth operation as follows.

15.4.2.1
Reduction of a Communication Amount of Data

The size of the image is switched to the 320 × 240-pixel format to reduce the amount of image data. In the case of the 320 × 240-pixel format, for obtaining an image-refreshing rate of five frames per second, it is possible to transfer one-quarter of the total image data by using a data transfer rate of 1 Mbps or less. Consequently, an adequate image-refreshing rate can be obtained, even when the line is congested. In such a case, when performing adjustment using the image including focusing, it is possible to reduce the size of image, to carry out the adjustment, and then to observe the image in an enlarged form. However, making picture size small has a limit. In this case, operability can be improved not only by changing the image size but also by changing the operation method.

15.4.2.2
Single-Action Operation

When sufficient refresh rate of an image is not obtained, stage movement and the continuous operations, such as focal adjustment, become impossible. The operation of stage movement is most influenced by the delay of the refresh speed of an image (Fig. 15.8). When moving a place of observation to the center of an image, in order to stop the stage moved to continuation in the target position, the refresh rate of image must be quick and must look continuous.

If the refresh rate of an image becomes slow, it is difficult to stop in the target position. In this case, when moving the stage, specify the target position on the screen on the client PC, as shown in Fig. 15.9, and then move the specified

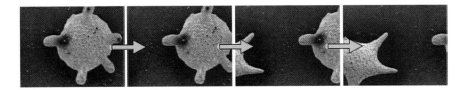

Fig. 15.8. Indication of image during the stage movement. When the refresh speed of the image is slow, (1) the image makes the frame movement, but (2) operator cannot stop the object position

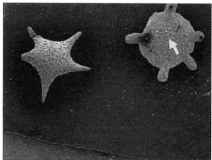
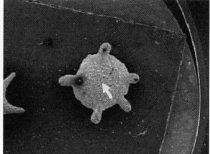

1)Click on the position to be moved   **2)The image moves to the center of the screen**

Fig. 15.9. Stage movement. Click the image position, indicated by arrow, then the image moves automatically to the center of the screen. When the network traffic is heavy, the stage position can be moved with certainty to the center of screen

position to the center of the image. This operation does not depend on the image-refreshing rate or the response to the control signal and enables the target position to be moved to the image center without fail. Therefore, it allows the image to be observed at a different magnification as soon as the target position has been moved. In addition, the use of automated functions such as autofocus, and autocontrast and brightness is useful for smooth operation. As shown here, the use of a complete single-action operation instead of a continuous operation is extremely effective for the congested line. For the remote, a further refinement for the complete single-action operation method, which is not based on the conventional SEM operation method, will make it possible to perform the remote operation using not only the LAN or Internet lines but also the network lines that cover a narrow band.

15.4.3
Case of the Operation of Remote Control

The case of the operation of remote control is shown below.

15.4.3.1
Difference in a Communication Method

As a method of using the communications network connected to the Internet, four systems are mainly used. As shown here, the difference of the communication method shows about influence for remote operation. The following four methods of connecting the remote control were used on this occasion.

To assess the practical applications of remote control, we connected an SEM located in Tokyo (JEOL):

1. ISDN (Integrated Services Digital Network: eight lines, approximately 1 Mbps). Connect from Fukuoka (Japan), 2001.
2. ADSL (asymmetric digital subscriber line: Measured value to the provider, approximately 3.6 Mbps). Connect from Osaka (Japan), 2002.
3. Internet (metal line). Connect from Seoul (Korea)/Boston (USA)/Adelaide (Australia), 2002.
4. Internet (optical line: FTTH 100 Mbps). Connect from Sapporo (Japan), 2007.

(1)–(3) were tested by WEB-SEM around 2002, (4) was tested by the remote desktop system in 2007. Figure 15.10 shows block diagram. The ISDN lines described in (1) are exclusive lines, and so these lines are not affected by external factors. The bandwidth of about 1 Mbps in the environment is always stabilized and can be connected. Consequently, as can be judged from the data transfer quantity indicated in Fig. 15.7, it is possible to perform adequately all the WEB-SEM operations by using a reduced screen.

In case of (2), ADSL is a communication line using a telephone wire (metal line). In the case of ADSL in (2), the data transfer speed to the Internet provider is about 3.6 MB/s. Therefore, this is an adequately high communication

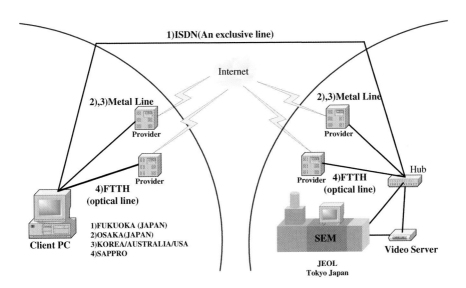

Fig. 15.10. Internet connection with Tokyo and the other places. (1) ISDN: 1 MB (eight lines), an exclusive line. (2) ADSL: 3.6 MB (effective value to provider), Internet connection. (3) Internet connection directory. (4) FTTH: optical line 100 MB

speed. However, this speed was greatly affected by the degree of congestion on the line between Osaka (provider) and Tokyo, and the communication speed was slightly less than that in ISDN. Also, the degree of congestion of the Internet connection varies greatly with the time; thus, depending on the particular time, the image-refreshing rate may fall to two or fewer images per second.

In the case of (3), the SEM is connected directly (metal line) to the Internet, and so the communication speed was greatly affected by the congestion and connection condition of the Internet. Because the transmission speed to a provider is quicker than ADSL of (2), it is thought that congestion or delay is produced on the Internet.

In (4), the optical line becomes popular from 2004. The optical circuit was used, and the connection test was done using the remote desktop system in 2007. An optical circuit (FTTH: fiber to the home) connected here has the communication capacity of 100 Mbps. And an optical line is steadier than a previously used metal line. The high-speed communication is achieved and, because the attenuation of the signal is little, data communication in a long distance is possible. SEM used JSM-7500F (made of JEOL) corresponding to a remote desktop method, and a remote system (PCAnywhereTM: made by the Symantec company) on the market was used for remote software. As a result, on the client PC screen, live image observation could be performed at the refresh speed of about four pictures per second. Although the remote desktop system needed large communication capacity for data transfer, SEM operation was possible at a lower capacity.

Compared with (2) or (3) measurement year, an optical line also spreads through the Internet network and the congestion during connection may be reduced.

15.4.3.2
Communication Channel and a Response

The communication environment at the time of using a global communications network is explained. In the case of (3), the SEM is connected directly to the Internet, and so the communication speed was greatly affected by the congestion and connection condition of the Internet. The connection using the Internet goes via two or more access points in a communication channel. As one of the causes, the response of each access point between SEM and client PCs is greatly related to delay of communication speed. The communication pass and response of access point were checked by the case where it connects to Japan (Tokyo) from South Korea (Seoul) of Fig. 15.10 (3). In this case, the Tracert command, which is a Dos command in Windows, was used. Table 15.1 shows the access points through which data pass between the client PC (within South Korea) and the basic unit of the SEM (in Japan), and also the response speed at each access point. The number in the left indicates the con-

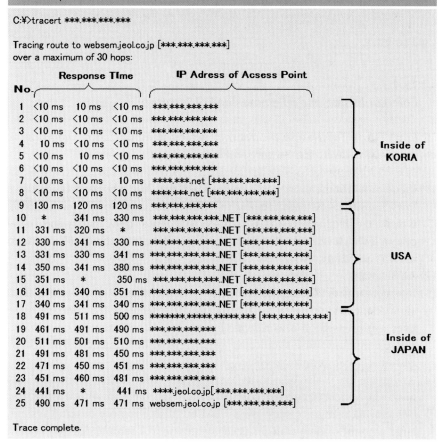

Table 15.1. The network environment when the Internet was connected from Seoul (South Korea) to Tokyo (JAPAN). The response speed was measured by using "tracert" command (DOS). Fully speed to the 9th access point for the communication (<10ms) can be obtained. But after 10th access point, the response speed became worse drastically (about 350ms), and the response speed became worse from 18th access point (about 500ms).

C:¥>tracert ***.***.***.***

Tracing route to websem.jeol.co.jp [***.***.***.***]
over a maximum of 30 hops:

	Response Time			IP Adress of Acsess Point	
No.					
1	<10 ms	10 ms	<10 ms	***.***.***.***	Inside of KORIA
2	<10 ms	<10 ms	<10 ms	***.***.***.***	
3	<10 ms	<10 ms	<10 ms	***.***.***.***	
4	10 ms	<10 ms	<10 ms	***.***.***.***	
5	<10 ms	10 ms	<10 ms	***.***.***.***	
6	<10 ms	<10 ms	<10 ms	***.***.***.***	
7	<10 ms	<10 ms	10 ms	****.***.net [***.***.***.***]	
8	<10 ms	<10 ms	<10 ms	****.***.net [***.***.***.***]	
9	130 ms	120 ms	120 ms	***.***.***.***	
10	*	341 ms	330 ms	***.***.***.***.NET [***.***.***.***]	USA
11	331 ms	320 ms	*	***.***.***.***.NET [***.***.***.***]	
12	330 ms	341 ms	330 ms	***.***.***.***.NET [***.***.***.***]	
13	331 ms	330 ms	341 ms	***.***.***.***.NET [***.***.***.***]	
14	350 ms	341 ms	380 ms	***.***.***.***.NET [***.***.***.***]	
15	351 ms	*	350 ms	***.***.***.***.NET [***.***.***.***]	
16	341 ms	340 ms	351 ms	***.***.***.***.NET [***.***.***.***]	
17	340 ms	341 ms	340 ms	***.***.***.***.NET [***.***.***.***]	
18	491 ms	511 ms	500 ms	*******.*****.*****.*** [***.***.***.***]	Inside of JAPAN
19	461 ms	491 ms	490 ms	***.***.***.***	
20	511 ms	501 ms	510 ms	***.***.***.***	
21	491 ms	481 ms	450 ms	***.***.***.***	
22	471 ms	450 ms	451 ms	***.***.***.***	
23	451 ms	460 ms	481 ms	***.***.***.***	
24	441 ms	*	441 ms	****.jeol.co.jp[.***.***.***.***]	
25	490 ms	471 ms	471 ms	websem.jeol.co.jp [***.***.***.***]	

Trace complete.

Note: IP address and a supplementary explanation are removed here.

nection sequence of the access point, and three of the time values to the right of it are the response times from the client PCs. At the access points 1–9, the response time of about not more than 10 ms was obtained within South Korea. The access points between 10 and 17 are connected to the USA. At the point where the route changes over from South Korea to the USA, the response time showed marked deterioration from 10 to about 350 ms. However, no deterioration of response was found at the access points within the USA. Access points 18–25 are located in Japan, and at the point of switching from the USA to Japan, the response deteriorates markedly. As can be seen from Table 15.1, there is no significant deterioration of response within each country and city, but a large deterioration occurs at the point bridging the two countries. The same phenomenon was also found in the case of Australia. The international connections made on this occasion were made directly between major cities in the countries concerned, and so the delay within each country was small. It was found that there was a delay at each international connection in this practical application. The communication is concentrated for the communication within a country. For this reason, communication speed gets worse among each country.

15.4.3.3
Communication and a Remote Control System

From the case of the operation shown earlier, communication and a remote control system have the following relations.

(1) ISDN provides the most stable environment because it consists of exclusive lines. However, because of the exclusive lines, the range to be used for ISDN is restricted. Furthermore, it is expensive to secure a large capacity line. In the case of ISDN, it is most suitable to secure the capacity of about 1 Mbps and to use a WEB-SEM system.

(2) ADSL and

(3) Internet are general-purpose lines, and so they are easy to use, but the operability depends greatly on the Internet environment. On the contrary, these lines can be used on a worldwide basis, and so they are very convenient. These communication should use WEB-SEM to be influenced by the congestion of a communication line.

(4) An optical line is also beginning to spread through ordinary homes quickly now. The optical circuit can connect a high-speed circuit of 100 Mbps. For this reason, using not only WEB-SEM but also a remote desktop system, large amount of data transfer is easily attained. A remote desktop system does not need the special tool and enables more users to use a remote desktop. In recent years, the optical line is used as the backbone of the Internet, and transmission speed is accelerated including the relay point. Thus, the spread of SEM on assumption of connection with the Internet and high-speed line enables it to share information simultaneously, more than before, between remote places. The optical line will be in use as the connection technique of remote control from now on, although it has not fully spread globally.

15.5
Conclusion

SEM has been effectively used in the field of biology and medicine until now. However, installation of SEM is limited to big universities, research centers, or hospitals because of the equipment size, expense associated with it, or lack of sample-treatment engineer. Establishment of a small hospital, etc., has not been realized till the present days. The scanning microscope has been used in limited area, because the information cannot be sent outside up to now. The remote control system of SEM can help in the precise diagnosis by providing the information acquired from a large magnification image to various medical specialists. Pathologist is able to connect simultaneously to two or more laboratories and hospitals, to specifically use the live image of SEM, and to point out a problem directly to a doctor. So far, remote control system has been shown to operate by one-to-one relation between an SEM and a client. Probably, it will also be required to distribute the same simultaneous image to two or more clients from now on. The teacher can show the live picture of an SEM to two or more students and impart special knowledge to them (Fig. 15.11). The students can learn by using a live image rather than looking at a photograph as found in textbook.

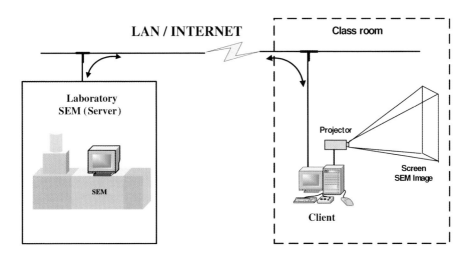

Fig. 15.11. Application example of WEB-SEM. By sharing the same information between the server side and the client side, mutual discussion using the live SEM image becomes possible

An SEM expands and observes the surface of a sample. The remote control system of SEM can help in observation at high magnification while moving the field of view from place to place, and not at a fixed place as in the photograph. Now, an optical line can also be developed in ordinary homes, and the Internet is becoming more accessible, which is cheap and can be easily connected. By connecting between clients with a direct optical line to SEM, the data transfer becomes high speed, and the response of each access point is also accelerated. Telepathology using an SEM will become possible anywhere in the world by being globally connected with a high-speed optical line from now on.

15.6
Summary

- In a pathology diagnosis, a pathologist uses not only an optical microscope but also a scanning electron microscope.
- An SEM operator and an observer at a remote place share the same information through the live image of a real sample at the same time.
- The SEM image transmits the image signal. The image signals are connected to the video server, and the image is transferred from the video server to the client PC via the LAN. Finally, the transferred images are displayed on the Internet explorer.
- The remote control properties of the SEM can be used for academic training and for communication between a laboratory and a factory, besides telepathology.
- However, installation of SEM is limited to big universities, research centers, or hospitals because of the equipment size, expense associated with it, or lack of sample-treatment engineer.

Telepathology: An Audit

Sajeesh Kumar

16.1
Telepathology is Advancing

Telepathology is a relatively young medical technology; consequently, further long-term studies with regard to patient advantages, cost effectiveness, and safety are required before the technology can be integrated into the mainstream health-care system. Telepathology services are not going away, but the field is changing. As with many young industries, telepathology seems to redefine itself on a fairly regular basis – changing to meet the demand of managing more and larger diagnostic images. The market is growing worldwide annually, due, in large part, to the approval of procedures. In addition, given better acceptance in the general marketplace among pathologists, surgeons, hospitals, and patients, this growth will likely increase. It must be noted that the growth of imaging technology and telecommunication technology will directly support and help the growth of telepathology, because these are, of course, an integral part of telepathology.

16.2
Will Telepathology Replace Traditional Methods?

Telepathology promises to revolutionize health care and speed the health-care process. Yet, the technology requires a great deal of further development. The introduction of telepathology does not mean that pathologists can abandon traditional methods. As well, the economics of telepathology must be further analyzed. Institutions must ensure that the cost of telepathology does not exceed the traditional expenses involved with pathology.

16.3
Issues Related to Telepathology: A Brief Overview

Immediate or widespread implementation of telepathology is hindered by many factors. The two biggest ones to be sorted out are the status of overseas reading of images and the evolving role of the virtual pathology department. Issues such as interpretation quality, reimbursement, and security are still in flux.

Issues related to telepathology may also include lack of telecommunication infrastructure, affordability of programs, cost of the equipments, accuracy of the medical and nonmedical devices used, training of personnel involved, lack of guidelines and protocols, sustainability of the projects, regulations regarding sharing of information, privacy, and legal liability.

16.4
Changing Industry

While the location issue needs to be resolved, the nature of telepathology services holds greater long-term impact on the future of pathology practice. What will telepathology practice look like in the coming years? To what extent and when might telepathology replace on-site pathologists?

Telepathology is driven by the relative shortage of pathologists and rising number of images to be interpreted – not the enabling technology. For the foreseeable future, getting all the images read will be the issue, not a competition between telepathology organizations and traditional groups.

The reality is that the local pathologist has much control of this situation. The local pathologist has the existing long-term community relationships and the ability to do procedures, on-site consultations, and conferences, as well as medical oversight in the pathology department. Most local pathology groups have exclusive contracts with the hospitals. Pathology groups choose to do business with telepathology companies with reputations, which they can trust. The biggest risk that a local pathology group can take is to continue in a seriously understaffed situation. By partnering with a trusted telepathology provider, they should find that their local hospital contract is more secure than it ever has been. Anything that improves service in the local practice will, in the form of better staffing levels, make it much harder for an outsider to compete.

If hospitals and groups have an on-site option, they are going to take it. Even sites with pathology groups in place are looking for someone to handle the overflow. A pathology group might read for five or six hospitals and use telepathology to shift work among its members. It may also contract with a telepathology company to handle overflow. Expansion may come in #dayside telepathology, because that is simply when most studies are being done. Of course, physicians' turnaround expectations are getting shorter, not longer.

16.5
Technical Challenge

One technical challenge to telepathology's dayside expansion is the availability of patients' prior examination and other data. Efficiently linking telepathology providers to patients' priors is an important step toward replicating the service of in-house pathology through telepathology. Of course, it requires that the originating hospital have IT systems in place to provide the information. Implementing this access could be the next quantum step in telepathology development.

16.6
Money Matters

Meeting the demand is a major telepathology driver, along with economic motivation. A group already large enough to staff and share off-hour call may show an economic benefit. Given imaging demand, pathologist lifestyle, and economic factors, telepathology services are not going away, but the field is rapidly changing. Besides quality pathologists, a track record of adaptability might be the trait facilities, and groups need to focus on when they consider implementing telepathology technology.

Financial planning for telepathology should include the costs of telecommunication and information technology infrastructure and medical devices, as well as costs such as personnel training, monthly network access fees, maintenance, telephone bills, and other operational expenses.

Once the objectives of a program are identified, technology support personnel should be consulted to clarify technical equipment specifications and facility requirements. Protocols and guidelines must be developed, which will provide clear direction on how to utilize telepathology most effectively. The training of operators is especially critical in telepathology. The reliability of a program is also related to the experience with telepathology technology and the awareness of its limitations.

Many nations do not have explicit policies to pay for telepathology services. A major telepathology payment policy is crucial. Meanwhile, several telemedicine services are being integrated to regular health-care systems in the USA and the Scandinavian countries with reimbursement/payment options. Studies should be conducted to implement, monitor, evaluate, and refine the telepathology payment process. Additionally, it should be noted that telepathology licensure and indemnity laws might also need to be formulated. This issue, however, remains a cloudy region for health-care strategists and has implications for pathologists and remote practitioners who practice across state or country lines.

It is observed that successful telepathology programs are often the product of careful planning, sound management, dedicated professionals and support staff, and a commitment to appropriate funding to support capital purchases and ongoing operations. It reflects a commitment to teamwork to link technical and operational complexities into a fully integrated and efficiently functioning program. Telepathology service providers, health insurance agencies, and all concerned institutions could convene to lead a workable model for telepathology service improvements. The professional communities could bring out telepathology service guidelines, which would pave the way for consensus on several difficult issues, including technical and service standardization for telepathology.

16.7
Conclusion

Health-care providers are now looking at telepathology as a model of improving, automating, and enhancing patient care. This book elaborates on many aspects of telepathology. Authors have shown telepathology to be practical, safe, and effective. Success often relates to the efficiency and effectiveness of the transfer of information and translates to improved or enhanced patient care than would otherwise be possible.

Available telepathology technology still has considerable room for improvement. However, the challenge is why, where, and how to implement which technology and at what costs. Asking the right questions will drive the technologies. A needs assessment is critical before implementing a telepathology project. Telepathology, as delineated in these pages, may appear novel but is rapidly coming into common and mundane usage through multiple applications. Time alone will tell whether telepathology (to paraphrase Neil Armstrong) is "one small step for Information & Communication Technology but one giant leap for pathology." However, from the pages of this first ever book on telepathology, the future promises to be exciting. Optimistically, the journey toward improved patient care will be well worth the wait for those benefiting from these technologies.

Glossary

Annotation of digital images   A process whereby images are marked or labeled electronically to identify specific features.

CADASIL   A rare inherited neurologic disease of young adults that can be diagnosed on skin samples by electron microscopy.

Consensus diagnosis   Arises in situations in which several experts contribute their opinions about the relative merits of a series of competing hypothesis.

CT   Used to guide fine needles into areas of pathology in a patient so that cells can be examined to help make a diagnosis by pathologists.

Cytologic smear   Refers to smears of cells applied to a microscopic slide that are viewed under a microscope.

Digital or virtual microscopy   A term describing the technology of preparing, handling, visualizing, archiving, and distributing "virtual slides." They can be diagnosed at local hospital, but also by many distant experts simultaneously, saving time and transportation costs. Virtual microscopy in combination with the emerging grid technology opens a new dimension for work sharing and scientific cooperation and will cause a paradigm shift in future pathology diagnostic practice.

Digital or virtual slide   The visual content of a conventional microscopic glass slide transferred into an equivalent computerized digital data set. Modern robotic microscopes or "scanners," depending on the section size on the original glass slide and requested optical magnification, need minutes to hours for production of a virtual slide. The result is a digital "big picture" file consisting of a matrix of electronically stitched "image tiles" captured from the original glass slide. The virtual slide offers a number of features not inherent in a glass slide. The "digital slide" can be visualized by a special viewer software program (mostly mimicking the functionality of a normal microscope) on a computer monitor and is called "virtual microscope."

DNA   The carrier of the genetic information (genotype) of each living organism, located mainly in the cell nucleus.

DNA ploidy analysis   A method that measures the DNA content within tumor cells.

Dynamic (active) telepathology system   Real-time, continuous movie-like image transfer from a microscope for diagnostic purposes. The consulting expert actively operates the distant-located microscope and chooses such operating parameters as specimen area and magnification, for observation.

eHealth   A term applied for health-care practice supported by electronic processes, informatics, and communication technology.

EM rapid virus diagnostic   Samples prepared with the negative-staining method can be diagnosed within half an hour. The method delivers clinically relevant diagnoses based on the morphology and size of the observed particles, which are characteristic for each virus family.

eScience   A term applied for computationally intensive science, which uses huge data sets and therefore requires grid computing.

Fine-needle aspiration cytology   A diagnostic technique in which a thin, hollow needle is inserted into the mass to extract cells that will be examined under a microscope.

Fluorescent in situ hybridization (FISH)   A cytogenetic method for detection and localization of presence or absence of specific DNA sequences on chromosomes using fluorescent probes binding specifically to diagnostic relevant sequences. A number of tumors display characteristic features in the DNA, which can be used for diagnostic purposes.

Frozen-section service   A pathological diagnostic procedure to obtain a rapid microscopic diagnosis by examining cryosections of intraoperative surgical tissue excisions. The mostly crude "benign" or "malignant" diagnosis provides important advice for the surgeon, determining the course and extent of patients' treatment.

G7SP4 conference   7th International telemedicine conference of the G7 Global Healthcare Application Sub-Project 4, held in Regensburg, September 22–25, 2002.

Genotype   The genotype describes the genetic constitution of an organism and is based on the inheritable genetic information coded in the DNA (mainly located in the cell nucleus). Genotype alterations can result in different disorders. Special genotypic assays including PCR techniques are suitable for analyzing the genotype status.

Grid technology   A new art of distributed or parallel computing in cyberspace using the Internet as a communication layer between the geographically disseminated dynamic "nodes" consisting of local computer clusters, dedicated instruments, information resources, and services. Integration of dynamic telemicroscopy and virtual microscopy systems opens new dimensions in medical service and cooperation.

H&E stain   Hematoxylin and eosin stain, used as standard staining method for thin tissue sections mounted on a glass slide and subjected to light microscopy pathologic examination.

HDSF   A telepathology system which can send both (hence the term "hybrid") dynamic (live) images and static (still) images. The still images tend to have much greater resolution than do dynamic images.

Histological section   Refers to thin slices of tissue applied to a microscopic slide, which are viewed under a microscope.

Immunohistochemical assay   Refers to the process of localizing proteins in cells of a tissue section exploiting the principle of antibodies binding specifically to antigens in biological tissues.

Immunohistochemistry   A microscopic technique to localize proteins (antibodies) in cells and tissue sections. Some of these are specific "markers" for a number of neoplasms and have a significant diagnostic value.

iTEM   A software package used in the described ultrastructural telepathology system (OSIS, Muenster, Germany)

"Live image" mode   Real-time, video-like image transfer from the sending server to the client (distant expert) during the telemicroscopic sample observation; used mostly in the search mode to find the diagnostically adequate sample area or objects.

Microwave-assisted tissue embedding For electron microscopic examination, the sampled tissue must be fixed, dehydrated in graded alcohol, and embedded in resin for cutting ultrathin sections. The turnaround time of this procedure (3–4 days) can be significantly reduced through the additional use of microwave energy during the different steps of the sample processing (4–6 h).

Miniaturized microscope array A technology for ultrarapid scanning of microscopic glass slides based on an ensemble of arrays of integrated mini lenses, parallel image processing of the captured images, and image reconstruction software. Currently, it is the last breakthrough in diagnostic virtual slide technology and has a significant impact on the developing virtual microscopy technique.

Mutation Changes in the base pair sequence of the DNA, which constitutes the genetic material of an organism. They can be the result of copying errors in the genetic material during cell division, but also caused by exposure to ultraviolet or ionizing radiation, chemical mutagenesis, or viruses.

Negative-staining method A rapid qualitative preparation method of virus suspensions (molecular aggregates) for electron microscopic examination. The observed virus particles are surrounded by a deposit of a heavy metal (1% uranyl acetate) from a dried solution, which creates a dark background in the EM image due to strongly scattered electrons; the particles themselves are displayed white (negative contrast).

NFD/NSF First described in 2000, systemic fibrosing disease, observed mainly in patients with renal insufficiency with a history of exposure to gadolinium-containing contrast agents (widely used for diagnostic magnetic resonance imaging).

Passive (static) telepathology Uses telecommunication technology for transfer of microscopic image sets captured by the sender for consultation to a distant expert. The expert must trust the sender that the right sample area and microscope magnification were chosen, to render a second-opinion diagnosis.

Phenotype Basically refers to the observed appearance (also microscopic morphology) of an organism and is the effect of the inherited genetic information coded in the DNA, located mostly in the cell nucleus. The phenotype is not simply a product of the genotype; it can be influenced by the environment and disease.

Polymerase chain reaction   A technique used in molecular biology for amplification of DNA pieces by enzymatic replication. Important for the detection and diagnosis of hereditary diseases and infectious agents.

POP   Access point to the wide area network.

Primary diagnosis   The number one working diagnosis.

Proficiency testing   A standardized test to evaluate and certify the quality of analysis.

Real-time telepathology   Synchronous form of telepathology in which the distant operator is able to command a distant robotized microscope by using software simulating the behavior of a microscope.

Reproducibility   Refers to the ability of a test or experiment to be accurately reproduced or replicated. It may be evaluated at the level of two or more observers examining the same specimen (interobserver reproducibility) or at the level of the same observer examining a specimen via two or more modalities or on two or more occasions (intraobserver reproducibility). It is measured by the k statistic.

"Same-day" diagnosis   Means diagnosis in a very short period of time, in which the pathological diagnosis is signed out on the day of receipt of the sample.

SBS-3Comsat satellite   Satellite Business System company, which launched their third commercial telecommunication satellite using the NASA Space Shuttle Columbia (STS-5) Mission on November 11, 1982. Installed in an operational geosynchronous orbit, no longer in service.

Second opinion   The opinion or interpretation of another (pathology) expert examining the same sample.

"Snapshot" image   Mostly captured at the end of the "live image" mode, the full-resolution 16-bit image transmitted from sender to the client (distant expert) during the telemicroscopic sample observation for storage in the local computer memory. Different discussion tools (arrow pointers, drawings, and annotations) and measurements can be synchronized between both sites, enhancing the telepresence effect.

Static image telepathology   Involves the capture of still digital images at one site and their electronic transmission and viewing at a distant site.

Store-and-forward telepathology   Form of telepathology based on the asynchronous exchange of either still images selected from a glass slide or a whole digital slide (although the latter case is usually referred as whole slide imaging).

Telediagnosis center   Specialized server system for telepathological second-opinion consultation of difficult diagnostic cases.

Telemedicine   A discipline of telematics (the combination of telecommunication and informatics technology), basically refers to the performance of a clinical medical service at a distance.

Telepathology   The practice of pathology through visualization of images indirectly on a computer monitor and usually entails electronic transmission of the images to a remote site. A discipline of telemedicine, a diagnostic pathology service at a distance, can be applied to light and electron microscopy. Now performed with passive (still image), active (live images, dynamic and interactive), hybrid, or virtual microscopy systems.

Telepresence microscopy   A technology that allows psychologically "to delete" the distance, separating two (or more) observers from each other during a microscopic sample examination. This is possible through the same sensual stimuli (vision and hearing) affected by the direct and distant-located observer (the same microscopic image visible on both monitors) and parallel voice communication. The "telepresence" feeling can be markedly increased using discussion tools synchronized between both displays and giving the distant operator nearly the same microscope operation functionality as the direct operator.

Teleradiology   A discipline of telemedicine, basically refers to electronic transmission of radiological patient images from one location to another (in the hospital and/or worldwide) for the purpose of interpretation and/or consultation.

Tissue-based diagnosis   A pathological expertise based mainly on the microscopic (light and/or electron) examination of diseased tissue or organs to clarify the nature of the lesion and give advice to the clinician for further patient treatment.

Tissue microarray   A paraffin block containing some hundreds of separate tissue cores assembled in array fashion for simultaneous histopathological analysis.

Ultrapath   Biannual Conference of the Society for Ultrastructural Pathology.

Ultrastructural telepathology   A procedure using a remotely live-operated electron microscope equipped with a digital camera for real-time, movie-like image transfer to a distant-located expert, for direct diagnostic purposes on the subcellular level of the sample. The specifically-for-collaboration tied-up software handles the connection via the Internet to the distant expert and gives him/her the same EM control as the observer sitting in front of the instrument has.

VAMC   A hospital and the associated grounds and building within the VHA.

VHA   That branch of the United States Department of Veterans Affairs which provides medical services to veterans through the administration and operation of numerous hospitals, medical centers, and outpatient clinics.

VISN   Groups of 6–12 Veterans Affairs Medical Centers in a geographic region that comprise one of 21 health-care networks in the VHA.

WAN   Computer network that covers a large area.

WSI   Technique based on the acquisition and visualization of digital slides.

Subject Index

Printing: Krips bv, Meppel, The Netherlands
Binding: Stürtz, Würzburg, Germany